This comprehensive resource describes every aspect of celiac disease including diagnosis and daily survival skills. There is an entire chapter which contains invaluable advice from those with the most experience—people with celiac disease!
—Trisha B. Lyons, RD, LD
MetroHealth Medical Center,
Cleveland, OH

A clear and comprehensive guide for anyone newly diagnosed with celiac disease, complete with valuable resources.
—Glutenfreeda.com, Inc.
(Jessica Hale and Yvonne Gifford,
Editors)

An excellent resource for those dealing with celiac disease and also for those who care for people with the disease. An invaluable tool with loads of resources and useful information presented in a concise, easy-to-understand manner!
—Marla Doersch, RD

A wonderfully comprehensive and invaluable guide to celiac disease, complete with the collective wisdom of the celiac community.
—Bonnie J. Kruszka,
Author of *Eating Gluten-Free with Emily*

This book will be a useful resource for those on gluten-free diets.
—Carol Fenster, Ph.D.,
Author of *Gluten-Free 101*

Kimberly Tessmer, RD, LD, has authoritatively compiled a wealth of useful information on the most life-altering aspect of celiac disease: its treatment. The highly practical and detailed information contained in this book will help both the celiac patient/parent and their healthcare providers minimize the bewilderment associated with following a gluten-free diet in today's fast-paced, fast-food, highly processed world.

—Kenneth Fine, M.D.
Founder and Director of EneroLab.com
Clinical Laboratory and the Intestinal
Health Institute, Dallas, Texas

This book is full of practical and helpful information on gluten-free living along with valuable tips and recipes from the experts themselves: those with celiac disease. This book would be a welcome addition to the celiac bookshelf!

—Shelley Case, B.Sc., RD
Author of *Gluten-Free Diet: A
Comprehensive Resource Guide*

Gluten-Free for a Healthy Life *covers the territory for those looking for information on celiac disease and the gluten-free diet.*

—Ann Whelan
Editor of *Gluten Free Living*

Gluten-free
for a
Healthy
Life

NUTRITIONAL ADVICE AND RECIPES FOR THOSE SUFFERING FROM CELIAC DISEASE AND OTHER GLUTEN-RELATED DISORDERS

Kimberly A. Tessmer, RD, LD

 NEW PAGE BOOKS
A division of The Career Press, Inc.
Franklin Lakes, NJ

GLUTEN-FREE FOR A HEALTHY LIFE
EDITED BY KATE HENCHES
TYPESET BY EILEEN DOW MUNSON
Cover design by Dorothy Wachtenheim
Printed in the U.S.A. by Book-mart Press

To order this title, please call toll-free 1-800-CAREER-1 (NJ and Canada: 201-848-0310) to order using VISA or MasterCard, or for further information on books from Career Press.

 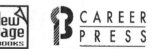

The Career Press, Inc., 3 Tice Road, PO Box 687,
Franklin Lakes, NJ 07417
www.careerpress.com
www.newpagebooks.com

Library of Congress Cataloging-in-Publication Data

Tessmer, Kimberly A.
    Gluten-free for a healthy life : nutritional advice and recipes for those suffering
    from celiac disease and other gluten-related disorders / by Kimberly A. Tessmer.
        p. cm.
    Includes index.
    ISBN 1-56414-688-X (pbk.)
        1. Gluten-free diet. 2. Gluten-free diet—Recipes. I. Title.

RM237.86.T47 2003
641.5'638—dc21

                                                                    2003044571

Disclaimer

At the time this book was written all information in this book was believed by the author to be correct and factual. Information on celiac disease and gluten-free food changes frequently as more research is being completed. Always keep yourself up-to-date by reading current publications and continue to check food ingredient lists. The author shall have no liability of any kind for damages of any nature however caused. The author will not accept any responsibility for any omissions, misinterpretations, or misstatements that may exist within this book. The author does not endorse any product or company listed in this book. The author is not engaged in rendering medical services and this book should not be construed as medical advice, nor should it take the place of regular scheduled appointments with your physician and/or dietitian. Please, consult your healthcare professional for medical advice.

To my Mom and Dad,
Don and Nancy Bradford,
who were role models teaching me that
anything is possible.
They passed on to me their knack for helping others
and have shown me, in the past few months, how
important it is to be there for people
and to take care of each other.
Thank you for all the love and encouragement you
have shown me throughout my life.

To my husband, Greg Tessmer, and my entire
family for their constant love, support, and
encouragement.

I would like to sincerely thank—

all of the people who helped me in so many ways to write this book. A very grateful thank you to all of the people with celiac disease who shared their time, ideas, tips, stories, and recipes with the hope of helping others.

Trisha Lyons, RD, LD, and Regina Celano: A very special thank you to both of you for all of your time and input into this book. Thank you for showing me the resilient, passionate, and caring spirit that people with celiac disease possess!

Many thanks also to: Shelley Case, B. Sc., RD, author of *Gluten-Free Diet: A Comprehensive Resource Guide*; Ann Whelan, editor of *Gluten Free Living*; Carol Fenster, Ph.D., Savory Palate, Inc., author of *Gluten-Free 101: Easy, Basic*

Dishes without Wheat; Yvonne Gifford, Editor & Chef of *Glutenfreeda* online cooking magazine; Jessica Hale, Editor & Chef of *Glutenfeeda* online cooking magazine; Kenneth Fine, M.D. of EnteroLab; Marla Doersch, RD; Bonnie Kruszka, author of *Eating Gluten-free with Emily*; Connie Sarros, author of *Wheat-free Gluten-free Cookbook for Kids and Busy Adults*; Bette Hagman, author of *The Gluten-Free Gourmet Cooks Fast and Healthy*; Christine A. Krahling, Communications Consultant; Lindsay Amadeo; Marcy Thorner of The Grammer Guru.

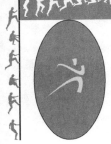

Table of Contents

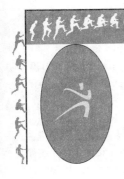

Introduction:
A Look Inside *Gluten-free for a Healthy Life*

Celiac disease has many names, such as gluten intolerance, gluten-sensitive enteropathy, and non-tropical sprue. Each name depicts a life-long autoimmune disorder in which a person's body cannot tolerate a group of grain proteins known as *gluten*. These grains consist of wheat, rye, barley, and any derivatives of these grains. Oats were always part if this list, but recent studies have shown that a moderate consumption of oats is safe for healthy children and adults who are well-established on a gluten-free diet. However, further studies are needed to determine long-term safety and contamination issues; therefore oats are not yet recommended by celiac organizations in the United States and Canada. Celiac disease was once thought to be rare, but is slowly being recognized as one of the most prevalent genetic disorders in the United States.

The only definite treatment for celiac disease is strict adherence to a 100-percent gluten-free diet for life. Learning and following a gluten-free diet are not easy tasks but can help prevent complications and symptoms that are associated with this disease. People with celiac disease need help in getting started in managing their diets and their lives and, through this book, I hope to provide enough practical information to do just that.

The good news is that people with celiac disease are not alone. There are all types of groups that provide resources and support for people with celiac disease and for their families. As the recognition of this disease grows, so does the pool of resources. There are more choices today than ever before for people with celiac disease.

This book serves many purposes. It will help people who have been clinically diagnosed understand what celiac disease is and the complex diet therapy that treats it. It is meant to help those who have the disease (and their families) learn how to manage their diet to lead a more comfortable, normal, and healthy life. Physicians, nurses, dietitians, chefs, food service staff, and other healthcare professionals may also find this source useful as they come in contact with people who suffer from celiac disease. This book also contains stories, tips, ideas, and recipes from people who have celiac disease. My hope is that people with celiac disease will feel more connected, touched, and inspired by others who share in their difficulty.

This book should not substitute a visit to a physician and/or dietitian who specializes in celiac disease and gluten-free diets. It should also not be used as your solitary means of treating your disease. Instead, the book should be used as a complement to their instruction and as a reference when needed.

Summing Up
Celiac Disease

Who Needs to Follow a Gluten-free Diet?

Celiac disease is one of the most prevalent reasons for a person to follow a gluten-free diet. Celiac disease is an autoimmune inflammatory disorder of the small intestine that is also known as gluten-sensitive enteropathy or non-tropical sprue. This disease can affect both children and adults. Its exact cause is unknown though recent research suggests that genetics is a strong component. Researchers believe that there are several genes that work together to cause celiac disease as opposed to a single missing or altered gene. Because our immune system is partly controlled by heredity, it goes without saying that celiac disease has a strong chance of running in the family.

For people with celiac disease, eating any food that contains gluten, a protein found in wheat, rye, barley, and any derivative of these grains, sets off an autoimmune response that causes the destruction of the villi within the lining of the small intestines as well as the destruction of digestive enzymes. Their body produces antibodies that attack the small intestines, causing damage and illness. Oats have also been traditionally considered to be harmful to people with celiac disease, but recent scientific studies have shown otherwise. (See Chapter 2 for more on oats.) The destruction of the villi results in the body's inability to absorb nutrients that are needed for good health, such as carbohydrates, protein, fat, vitamins, and minerals. These nutritional deficiencies can deprive the brain, nervous system, bones, liver, heart, and other organs of the nourishment they need and cause vitamin and mineral deficiencies leading to many types of illnesses. Celiac disease is not curable and there are currently no drugs to treat it. The only form of treatment is strict adherence to a 100-percent gluten-free diet for life. Once on a gluten-free diet, symptoms will diminish and the small intestines will heal and return to normal.

Gluten-free diets are also used to treat *dermatitis herpetiformis* (DH). DH is a chronic and severe disease of the skin that presents itself with itchy skin blisters on the elbows, knees, buttocks, scalp, and back. DH is also a genetic autoimmune disease and is linked to celiac disease, though both are separate diseases. In fact, about 5 percent of people with celiac disease will develop DH, either before being diagnosed or within the first year on the diet. When a person with DH consumes gluten, it triggers an immune system response that deposits a substance, immunoglobulin gamma A (IgA), under the top layer of the skin. Once the IgA is deposited under the skin, a gluten-free diet can slowly clear it. Most people with DH do not have obvious gastrointestinal symptoms, but almost all have some type of damage to the small intestines. Therefore they also have the potential for all of the nutritional problems of a person with celiac disease. Both celiac disease and DH are permanent. With both conditions, symptoms and damage will occur if gluten is consumed.

There are also people who suffer from a less aggressive form of gluten intolerance. General *gluten intolerance* is even harder to diagnose than celiac disease because there are no established diagnostic criterion. People who may have a general intolerance to gluten do not experience the severe symptoms that those who have celiac disease experience, but a gluten-free diet can substantially improve their health and quality of life.

Prevalence of Celiac Disease

New medical studies are indicating that celiac disease is much more common than once thought. According to one of the newest and largest studies performed to establish the prevalence of celiac disease in the United States (by the University of Maryland Center for Celiac Research, the University of Maryland School of Medicine, and other large medical entities, reported in the Archives of Internal Medicine) one out of every 133 people in the general population have celiac disease. This translates to 2.2 million Americans. This same research found that the presence of celiac disease in at-risk groups (people who either have celiac disease in the family or who have gastrointestinal symptoms) was one in 22 people in first-degree relatives, one in 39 people in second-degree relatives, and one in 56 people who had gastrointestinal symptoms or a disorder associated with celiac disease. The results of this newest study concluded that celiac disease does occur frequently in people with gastrointestinal symptoms as well as in first- and second-degree relatives of those that have the disease. The disease was as prevalent in first- and second-degree relatives *with* symptoms as it was in relatives *without* symptoms. This further emphasizes the existence of a family history of celiac disease as a risk factor. The study also found a high prevalence of celiac disease in people who had related health issues, such as Type 1 diabetes, anemia, arthritis, osteoporosis, infertility, and Down syndrome, even if these people did not show gastrointestinal symptoms.

Research has indicated that celiac disease is twice as common as Crohn's disease, ulcerative colitis, and cystic fibrosis combined. Celiac disease can show up at any age and can sometimes be triggered by events such as surgery, pregnancy, childbirth, viral infections, or severe emotional stress. Until recently, it was mostly recognized in children. The rate at which adults are being diagnosed is increasing rapidly thanks to greater awareness and improved diagnostic skills.

Though celiac disease has always been thought rare in the United States, it is one of the most common genetic diseases in many European countries. Because it is a genetic disease, researchers wonder why the disease is so uncommon in the United States when so many Americans are decedents from European groups. This may be because celiac symptoms mirror many other illnesses making it one of the most misdiagnosed diseases in the United States today. It may also be because physicians, and even registered dietitians, have always been taught that celiac disease is rare and that patients were only thought to have the disease if they had the classical gastrointestinal symptoms. The result of this mindset is that people are not routinely tested for celiac disease. Medical professionals now know that there are people who display no gastrointestinal symptoms despite having gluten sensitivity. Celiac disease may also be under-diagnosed due to the use of antibody blood tests that are not as specific as others or biopsy samples not taken from active patches of the disease. No matter what the reason, more research is needed to find out the true prevalence of celiac disease in the United States, and more education is needed to ensure that people with varying symptoms, other health conditions, or high-risk family histories are correctly and promptly screened.

What Are the Symptoms of Celiac Disease?

The range of symptoms associated with celiac disease ranges widely. There are really no "typical" symptoms because they vary so greatly from person to person, ranging from having no symptoms to suffering the most extreme symptoms. Many people with the disease are asymptomatic for years, becoming active only after something triggers it, such as surgery, viral infection, severe emotional stress, pregnancy, and/or childbirth. Research has discovered that symptoms of celiac disease not only appear in the gastrointestinal tract, but in the neurological, endocrine, orthopedic, reproductive, and hematological systems as well. It is essential to visit your physician if you have celiac disease symptoms for more than seven days or if you suspect that you have celiac disease *at all*. Both children and adults can experience one or more of the following symptoms:

- Reoccurring abdominal bloating and pain.
- Nausea and vomiting.
- Diarrhea.
- Weight loss.
- Iron deficiency with or without unexplained anemia.
- Vitamin and mineral deficiencies.
- Edema or excessive fluid retention.
- Chronic fatigue, weakness, and lack of energy.
- Pale and foul-smelling stool.
- Depression.
- Bone or joint pain.
- Muscle cramps.
- Constipation.
- Chronicly alternating diarrhea with constipation.
- Excessive flatulence.
- Balance problems.
- Migraine.
- Seizures or other neurological reactions.
- Memory problems.

Infants and children may also display additional symptoms:

- Growth failure to thrive.
- Bloated abdomens.
- Behavioral changes, including irritability.
- Growth and maturation problems.
- Learning challenges and disabilities.
- Dental enamel defects.

Because there can be a great length of time between the onset of symptoms and a diagnosis, there is a greater chance for nutritional deficiencies as well as lactose intolerance to develop. For people with celiac disease, lactose intolerance is more prevalent because the damage to the gastrointestinal tract can reduce the level of lactase in the body. Lactase is the enzyme needed to completely break down lactose (a natural sugar contained in milk and milk products). When lactose is not completely broken down a person may experience some or all of the following symptoms: gas, diarrhea, bloating, abdominal cramping, nausea, and headache. Lactose intolerance and the symptoms that accompany it are usually temporary until the celiac disease is under control and the small intestine heals.

Reactions (after eating gluten) can be immediate for some people or may be delayed for weeks or months for others. No two reactions are alike when it comes to celiac disease. But with total withdrawal of gluten from the diet, the result is disappearance of the symptoms associated with celiac disease.

The reason some people with celiac disease may not experience symptoms may be due to an undamaged part of their small intestines that is able to absorb enough nutrients to prevent the onset of these symptoms. They may not experience symptoms, but they are still at risk for the complications of celiac disease.

How Is Celiac Disease Diagnosed?

The task of diagnosing celiac disease is a difficult one because symptoms range widely along with their severity. Celiac disease is often misdiagnosed as irritable bowel syndrome, colitis, Crohn's disease, diverticulosis, intestinal infections, psychiatric complications, post-partum depression, and even chronic fatigue syndrome. In the United States, the average length of time from the start of symptoms and a confirmed diagnosis is 11 years. If your physician suspects celiac disease you should be referred to a gastroenterologist (a specialist in the areas of the stomach and intestines) who has experience with celiac disease. Keep in mind that a gastroenterologist is not the only type of doctor who may notice symptoms. Other specialized doctors such as endocrinologists, rheumatologists, OB/GYNs, and dermatologists may also take part in observing signs of celiac disease.

The first step in the diagnosis process is a simple blood test. Special types of blood antibody tests are used in screening for gluten intolerance. You are tested for the presence of these antibodies:

- ☐ Tissue Transglutaminase (tTG) IgA.

- ☐ Anti-endomysial Antibody (EMA) IgA.

- ☐ Anti-gliadin Antibody (AGA) IgA and IgG (immunoglobulin gamma G).

There are certain antibodies in the body that are produced by the immune system in response to substances that are perceived as threatening to the body. These particular antibodies are higher than normal in people with celiac disease who are consuming a diet that contains gluten. The levels of these antibodies tend to fall once a gluten-free diet has begun. If all three tests come back positive and the person has been eating a diet that contains gluten, there is a good chance the person has celiac disease. **A person should never follow a gluten-free diet before having blood tests (and/or a biopsy) done, because this can interfere with test results and therefore a correct diagnosis.** Often, mixed results will occur, which make the tests inconclusive. The blood antibody tests are not a definitive tool for diagnosing celiac disease. The *absence* of these antibodies does not guarantee a person *does not* have celiac disease, and the *presence* of them does not guarantee that a person *has* celiac disease.

If the blood tests along with symptoms suggest the probability of celiac disease, the next step would be a biopsy that would check for actual damage to the villi. A biopsy is the most conclusive test for celiac disease. An intestinal biopsy involves a long, thin tube, called an "endoscope." It is passed through the mouth and stomach and into the small intestines. The instrument is able to obtain a small sample of the villi or tissue of the small intestine. If damage to the villi is found the physician may place the person on a gluten-free diet for at least six months and then perform a second biopsy, to see if the lining has healed. Most physicians will accept a positive antibody test, one positive biopsy, and improvement of symptoms after a gluten-free diet as sufficient evidence for a positive diagnosis of celiac disease. Procedures will differ depending on your physician and his or her judgment.

To recap, a proper diagnosis for celiac disease should include the following steps:

1. A suspicion of celiac disease based on symptoms, physical appearance, and abnormal blood tests.

2. A small intestinal biopsy that shows damage to the villi.

3. Definite improvement with a total gluten-free diet.

Americans are not routinely screened or tested for the antibodies to gluten. However, because celiac disease is genetic, family members (especially immediate family of people who have been diagnosed) should be screened for the disease. That includes people who are asymptomatic. The longer a person with celiac disease goes undiagnosed and untreated, the greater his or her chances are of developing severe malnutrition and other health complications. It is also suggested that people who have other autoimmune disorders be screened for celiac disease.

How Is Celiac Disease Treated?

Completely eliminating gluten from the diet is the only known treatment for celiac disease. A gluten-free diet is essential for life. Following a gluten-free diet means avoiding any food products that contain wheat, rye, barley, and their derivatives. This means avoiding most starches, pasta, cereal, breads, and many processed foods that contain those grains. Once gluten is removed from the diet, the villi and tissues of the small intestine can begin to heal, and associated symptoms will begin to diminish. The National Institute of Diabetes and Digestive and Kidney Diseases (NIDDK) states, "For most people, following this diet will stop symptoms, heal existing intestinal damage, and prevent further damage. Improvements begin within days of starting the diet, and the small intestine is usually completely healed—meaning the villi are intact and working—in three to six months. (It may take up to two years for older adults.)"

A gluten-free diet must be followed for a *lifetime*, not just until the intestines are healed. Eating any amount of gluten can cause tissue damage, whether there are symptoms present or not. During the first few months of the gluten-free diet, or until the villi of the small intestines has healed, your physician may supplement your diet with vitamins and minerals to remedy any deficiencies and to replenish your nutrients. If lactose intolerance has developed, a lactose-free diet will also be necessary, though this often returns to normal within a few months of starting a gluten-free diet.

The diet of a person with celiac disease can be healthy, tasty, and well-balanced. The key is education. It is vital to learn how to read food labels and substitute foods that have wheat flour for foods such as potato, rice, corn, and soy. To make it a bit easier for people who must follow a gluten-free diet, there are many gluten-free products available from specialty food companies. A gluten-free diet can be a complicated one, and a person on a gluten-free diet must be extremely careful when eating at restaurants, buying lunch at school or work, eating at parties, grabbing food from a vending machine, or simply having a midnight snack. With the right education and with enough practice, living on a gluten-free diet can become second nature. It is vital to have the right attitude! *Accept your disease, educate yourself, and move on.* Don't let the disease control your life! Instead, control the disease and live a normal life. Seek professional guidance from a dietitian to help you get started in the right direction.

The most important aspects of treatment for a celiac involve:

- Maintaining strict adherence to a gluten-free diet for life.

- Learning all there is to know about the basics of following a gluten-free diet in order to self-manage your diet.

- Helping others in your life to understand the basics of a gluten-free diet.

- Adjusting to the diet to fit it into everyday life and making any adjustments necessary for other special needs beyond the gluten-free part of the diet.

- Adjusting for other potential needs related to blood test evaluations that include levels of vitamins and minerals.

- Evaluating bone mineral density with the appropriate follow-ups as indicated by your physician.

- Continuous monitoring by your physician to evaluate your progress and medical status as well as detect any changes in your condition that may call for additional treatment.

A Nutritional Gluten-free Diet

Following a gluten-free diet should not mean that you can no longer follow a healthy diet. Your main focus should still be to follow the Food Guide Pyramid and eat from *all* of the food groups each day. The key is to build your healthy eating plan using alternative grains. Foods with whole wheat flours such as breads, cereals, and pasta are great sources of complex carbohydrates, fiber, and nutrients such as B vitamins and iron. In the United States most refined wheat flours, wheat-based food products, and cereals are enriched with thiamin, riboflavin, niacin, folic acid, and iron. Unfortunately many of the gluten-free grain products are not enriched. Therefore many of the specially made gluten-free grain products may not provide the same amount of nutrients as their wheat-containing counterparts.

Because wheat is a large contributor of dietary fiber in an average diet and because many gluten-free foods are low in fiber, it is important to ensure that you consume the recommended amount of fiber daily. The U.S. Food and Nutrition Board recommends that adult men older than 50 years of age consume 30 grams daily and that adult women older than 50 years of age consume 21 grams. For adult men and women younger than 50 years of age the recommended intakes are 38 grams and 25 grams, respectively. Eat a variety of high-fiber, gluten-free foods daily such as fresh fruits, fresh vegetables, legumes, nuts, seeds, and brown rice. Higher-fiber gluten-free flours and grains include amaranth, cornmeal, flax seed, chickpea (garbanzo) flour, garfava flour, millet seeds, rice bran, and soy flour (defatted).

To help increase your intake of these B vitamins, iron, and fiber:

- Eat fresh fruits and vegetables often (at least five servings per day).

- Eat the edible skins of fruits and vegetables such as those of apples and potatoes. The skin contains most of the fiber in some produce.

- Choose *enriched* gluten-free products as often as possible.

- Choose whole-grain gluten-free products as opposed to refined, gluten-free grains. For example, use brown rice instead of white rice.

- Choose gluten-free products that incorporate higher nutritive gluten-free grains such as buckwheat, bean, quinoa, amaranth, and soy.

- Eat foods that are high in vitamin C with iron-rich foods to increase your absorption of iron.

- Drink coffee or tea between meals instead of with meals.

- Increase your intake of foods that are naturally gluten-free and are higher in the B vitamins and iron, such as lean meats, legumes, eggs, peanut butter, fish, dairy products, green leafy vegetables, brown rice, nuts (almonds), seeds (sunflower), fruit juices (orange and tomato), potatoes, and basically *all* other plant foods.

- Talk to your doctor about taking a daily gluten-free multi-vitamin/mineral supplement as well as a gluten-free calcium supplement. If you are not sure how much to take or what brand to use, contact your dietitian or physician.

Are There Complications of Celiac Disease?

Due to the damage in the small intestines and its inability to absorb nutrients, people with celiac disease are more likely to be afflicted with specific health problems if the disease goes untreated. These health problems can include:

- Osteoporosis/Osteopenia.
- Tooth enamel defects.
- Central and peripheral nervous system diseases.
- Pancreatic disease.
- Vitamin K deficiency associated with an increased risk for hemorrhaging.
- Disorders of the gallbladder, liver, or spleen.
- Gynecological disorders such as amenorrhea, miscarriages, and infertility.

People who have celiac disease who do not strictly adhere to a gluten-free diet have greater chances of developing cancer in the intestinal wall as well as other gastrointestinal areas. Some of the complications that accompany celiac disease can be healed or the risk lowered after adequate time on a gluten-free diet.

What Other Diseases/Disorders Are Linked With Celiac Disease?

There seems to be a higher occurrence of other diseases and disorders, many of them other autoimmune disorders, for people with celiac disease. The connection between celiac disease and some of these diseases/disorders may be strictly genetic.

Some of these diseases and disorders include:

- Dermatitis Herpetiformis (DH).
- Insulin-dependent Diabetes (Type 1).
- Thyroid disease.
- Sjogrens syndrome.
- Systemic Lupus Erythematosus.
- Rheumatoid arthritis.
- IgA nephropathy and IgA deficiency.
- Kidney disease.
- Carcinoma of the oropharynx, esophagus, and small bowel.
- Liver disease.
- Graves' disease.
- Addison's disease.
- Chronic active hepatitis.
- Scleroderma.
- Down syndrome.

Most recently it has been reported that a gluten-free diet may help other conditions such as autism, chronic fatigue syndrome, multiple sclerosis, and attention-deficit hyperactivity disorder. These findings are not yet proven, but more research is being conducted.

A gluten-free diet is not, by any means, a cure for any of these conditions, but it could offer relief for some. Talk to your healthcare provider about the possible benefits of a gluten-free diet for you.

Knowing that people with celiac disease have a greater incidence of certain health problems, emphasis should be put on seeing your physician for regular check-ups and taking care of your health.

Autism and Dietary Intervention

Some groups are now advocating protocol that recognizes prescribing a gluten-free, casein-free (free of a protein fraction found in dairy products) diet for at least three months to children who show autistic behavior. It may take at least a three-month trial period to actually determine if the diet makes a difference. There has recently been a theory that shows that the inability to break down certain foods (such as the proteins in gluten and casein) may affect the developing brain in some children, causing autistic behavior. These undigested, unbroken proteins (called peptides) are normally excreted in the urine though a few enter the bloodstream. Unbroken peptides that enter the bloodstream attach to the opiate receptors of the child's brain and seem to cause abnormal brain development and an opiate-like effect. (Opiates are highly addictive and can reach toxic levels.) The opiate-like effect can cause the child to feel drowsy, can block pain receptors, and can depress activity of the nervous system. A urine test can detect unbroken peptides. If high levels of the unbroken peptides show up in the urine it may be worth placing the child on a gluten-free, casein-free diet.

Research does not yet prove that a gluten-free, casein-free diet will help every child with autistic behaviors, but it is still being conducted. The diet must be all or nothing to actually determine if it makes a difference.

For More Information:

> Autism Society of America
> 7910 Woodmont Avenue, Suite 650
> Bethesda, Maryland 20814-3015
> Phone: (301) 657–0881   Fax: (301) 657–0869
> E-mail: info@autism-society.org

> Autism Network for Dietary Intervention (ANDI)
> Fax: (609) 737–8453
> E-mail: AutismNDI@aol.com

Communicating With Your Physician

Your first order of business is to find a physician that meets your needs. A specialist in the gastrointestinal area is called a gastroenterologist. Depending on your healthcare plan you may need to be referred to a specialist by your primary care provider. Your physician should be someone you completely trust and feel comfortable speaking with about concerns, suspicions, and feelings. Your physician should be someone who is open to any new information you have learned concerning celiac disease. Find a physician who allows you to actively participate in your own healthcare and who provides any support and assistance necessary to diagnose and treat your disease. Be sure that the physician you choose has adequate knowledge of celiac disease and is willing to screen patients for celiac disease.

It is a smart idea to keep copies of all your medical records, which you are legally entitled to. This keeps you more in control and up to date with your disease and treatment and it will also make it easier if you need to change doctors at any point. Be sure to schedule an exam every year along with any tests that are appropriate for your age and risk factors. It is important for people with celiac disease to have a gluten antibody test once a year to monitor their response to their gluten-free diet. A positive test would let you know that you need to follow your gluten-free diet a bit closer. Other annual screenings should include thyroid and blood tests to measure for folic acid, calcium, iron, and vitamins D, A, K, and B12. Bone density should also be tested annually for individuals who have abnormal results.

When choosing a specialist you can begin by consulting your primary care provider. A second information source could be your local county's medical societies. Another excellent route is to contact the state university medical center in your area. You can call and ask for a referral or a phone number for the chair of the department of gastroenterology. A state university medical center will make other specialty departments more accessible to you in case you need them, as well as provide you with a substantial medical team to monitor all aspects of your condition.

It is important to be prepared before you visit your doctor. Know what questions you are going to ask and write them down so you can't forget them. If you suspect you have celiac disease, do your homework and brush up on the basics before your visit. During your visit ask whatever questions you feel you need to and don't be intimidated! This is *your* health and *your* body, and you have the right to know and understand what is going on. Write down the answers to your questions and, if the doctor is not clear with an answer, speak up. Repeat the doctor's answers to verify that you understand. Be sure to let the doctor know if there are others in your family who have celiac disease or who experience the same type of symptoms that you do. Bring a friend or family member with you to help. Sometimes it helps to have at least two pairs of ears listening for better understanding and retention. Don't be rushed out of the doctor's office. Stay until you feel all of your questions have been answered and you fully understand your condition, diagnosis, treatment, and so forth. Before you leave the doctor's office make sure you know exactly how to contact the doctor for any follow-up questions that may arise. *Most importantly*, if you are not getting the results you want from your doctor or specialist, *seek the advice of another physician*. You have every right to get to the bottom of your symptoms and improve your health. Just because a physician is a gastroenterologist does not necessarily mean he or she specializes in celiac disease.

The following are some important questions to ask the physician, whether you suspect you may have celiac disease or if you have been diagnosed with celiac disease and are searching for a physician:

☐ What is your background and experience with celiac disease?

- ☐ How many patients with celiac disease have you seen in the last year?

- ☐ How rare or common is celiac disease?

- ☐ What causes celiac disease?

- ☐ Can you explain celiac disease, or gluten intolerance, and its symptoms?

- ☐ How is celiac disease diagnosed?

- ☐ How is celiac disease treated?

- ☐ Should my family members be screened for celiac disease if I have it?

- ☐ Is it okay to have some gluten in the diet?

- ☐ Should I take vitamin/mineral supplements?

- ☐ Could I have associated food intolerances?

- ☐ Why and where should I have a bone density test done?

- ☐ What other tests should I have done at the beginning and on a regular basis?

- ☐ What concerns should I have from celiac disease?

- ☐ What complications could I experience with celiac disease?

- ☐ Who can best teach me about a gluten-free diet?

Living With Celiac Disease

Living with celiac disease can be very challenging. However, as you learn more and more, managing your disease will get easier and become second nature. Use these suggestions to help you cope more easily:

- **Collect all the information you can about celiac disease and gluten-free diets.** Talk to your physician, search the Internet (make sure to stick with reputable Websites), read books and pamphlets, purchase specialized gluten-free cookbooks, and become familiar with gluten-free associations and groups. Knowledge is power. The more you know, the more control you have and the easier life with celiac disease will be.

- **Educate your loved ones.** As important as it is for *you* to know all about a gluten-free diet, it is just as important for your *spouse* and/or *family members* to understand the basics of the diet.

- **Don't go it alone!** Seek out others who have celiac disease and can help and support you through the tough times. There are plenty of local support groups as well as chat rooms and message boards on the Internet that can help provide all kinds of support.

- **Seek the guidance of a professional.** Getting started can be difficult and overwhelming, so don't hesitate to seek the guidance of a dietitian who specializes in celiac disease and gluten-free diets. A dietitian can help you sort through the foods you are allowed and not allowed and provide you with valuable information. You can contact the American Dietetic Association at *www.eatright.org* to find a dietitian in your area, or ask your physician to refer you to one. Keep in mind to choose a dietitian and physician who specialize in celiac disease and gluten-free diets.

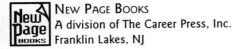

4 The Gluten-free Kitchen

Stocking Your Kitchen Cupboard

It is a great idea to clear out a special cupboard in the kitchen to store all the special products you will need for the gluten-free diet. Making sure you always have certain products on hand will make whipping up meals and snacks much easier. You can make things even easier by batch cooking. Cook large quantities of food or dishes and freeze the leftovers in individual storage containers to allow for a quick and easy meal or snack.

People on gluten-free diets often need to cook from scratch to ensure that meals and dishes are in fact gluten-free. Cooking from scratch does not have to be so time-consuming. There are several kitchen appliances you can use to help reduce your workload. Bread-makers, heavy-duty mixers, and pasta makers can be very helpful additions to the gluten-free kitchen.

As with any type of diet, it is wise to plan ahead when on a gluten-free diet. Having the following foods on hand will ensure no-hassle preparation when it is time for a meal or snack.

Gluten-free kitchen essentials:

- Assorted jams and jellies.
- Baking powder (gluten-free, such as Clabber Girl or Calumet).
- Baking soda.
- Beans: chickpeas, kidney beans, lentils, gluten-free refried beans, gluten-free baked beans.
- Breads: gluten-free bread, bagels, buns, waffles, and/or muffins.
- Bread crumbs (gluten-free).
- Bouillon base and cubes (gluten-free).
- Canned chicken.
- Canned tuna or salmon.
- Cereal (gluten-free), such as puffed rice, puffed corn, Corn Pops, cream of rice. *(Be careful of cereals that may be made from corn or rice but contain malt.)*
- Cheese.
- Chili with beans (gluten-free, such as Hormel).
- Condiments (relish, gluten-free ketchup, such as Heinz, mustard.)
- Cornstarch.
- Corn tortillas or tacos.
- Cottage cheese.
- Crackers (gluten-free).
- Cream of tartar.
- Eggs (whole, fresh).
- Flour: bean flour, chickpea flour, cornstarch, cornmeal, potato starch flour, brown/white rice flour, sorghum flour, soy flour, tapioca flour.
- Fresh and/or frozen fruit.
- Fresh meats (be careful of deli meats).
- Fresh and/or frozen vegetables.
- Fruit juices.
- Herbs and pure spices (such as garlic powder, onion powder, pure black pepper).
- Honey.
- Margarine or butter.
- Milk.
- Mixes for gluten-free bread, muffins, waffles, cakes, and brownies.
- Nuts and seeds.
- Onions.

- Pasta (gluten-free, such as rice, corn, potato, legume, quinoa).
- Peanut butter (gluten-free).
- Popcorn, plain or gluten-free microwave popcorn.
- Potatoes (whole).
- Rice (brown, white, or wild).
- Rice cakes: gluten-free mini flavored rice cakes or the large version.
- Salad dressings (gluten-free).
- Sauces (gluten-free): barbecue sauce, pizza sauce, pasta sauce, salsa, soy sauce, teriyaki sauce.
- Seeds and nuts (almonds, peanuts, walnuts, sunflower seeds, sesame seeds).
- Sugar (white and brown).
- Tofu.
- Tomato paste, whole tomatoes, diced tomatoes, tomato sauce (gluten-free).
- Vanilla.
- Vegetable oil.
- Vinegar: white and red wine, cider, rice and balsamic.
- Xanthan gum or guar gum.
- Yogurt: plain or gluten-free fruited yogurt, such as Yoplait.

All About Gluten-free Flours

There are plenty of gluten-free mixes on the market today that are perfect for breads, muffins, biscuits, cakes, and any of your favorite baked goods, but you can still bake from scratch if your heart so desires. It just takes a little extra work when baking with gluten-free flours. Many health-food stores, specialty online gluten-free stores, and possibly your local grocery store will sell gluten-free flours and/or mixes. There are many types of flours that are gluten-free, but the typical ones include corn, rice, soy, tapioca, potato starch flour, or a mixture of these. Using these types of flours in place of wheat flour may give foods a different taste and texture so practice and experiment with them to find the right combination. There are all types of cookbooks that can provide you with detailed information about gluten-free baking along with scrumptious recipes. (See Chapter 9.)

The following is a list of some of the types of gluten-free flours:

Amaranth: Mild nut-like flavor and good for baking, it is best when used in combination with other gluten-free flours.

Arrowroot flour: No real flavor, typically used as a thickener in many foods, similar in texture to cornstarch and can be exchanged for cornstarch measure for measure in recipes and mixes.

Brown rice flour: Slightly sweet, mild flavor, and excellent for use in desserts, it has a higher nutrient content (including fiber) than white rice flour and contains bran. Use it in combination with other gluten-free flours as a type of binding agent (such as eggs, mashed banana, or applesauce) to avoid a crumbly end product. Best used for breads, muffins, and cookies where a bran or nutty type flavor is desired. Due to the oils in the bran, this flour has a short shelf life and its flavor will become stronger as it ages. Purchase it fresh and store it in the refrigerator or freezer to preserve it longer.

White rice flour: Not much flavor or nutrition, it has a long shelf life, and is best used in combination with other gluten-free flours.

Buckwheat flour: Strong flavored, it's best when used in small quantities in combination with other gluten-free flours. Even though it has wheat in the name it is gluten-free and not related to wheat—it is instead related to the rhubarb plant. (Be aware that some companies mix buckwheat flour with wheat flour to lessen its strong taste).

Chickpea flour: Hearty but mild flavor, made from garbanzo beans, and high in protein and fiber, it can be used in combination with other gluten-free flours and when baking.

Corn flour: Milled from corn (maize), has a mild corn taste, and adds a light texture to baked goods, it is great for blending with cornmeal to make corn bread for corn muffins and best when used in combination with other gluten-free flours.

Garfava flour: A blend of garbanzo and fava beans, developed by Authentic Foods, it is high in protein and fiber, and it creates excellent volume and moisture content in baked goods.

Millet flour: Because it tends to make breads dry and course, substitute only 1/5 of the flour mixture with this flour.

Nut or legume flours:
Nutty in flavor, it can be used in small portions to enhance the taste of puddings, cookies, or homemade pasta.

Potato flour: Not the same as potato starch flour and heavier in texture, it is best when used in small quantities and combined with other gluten-free flours, and should be stored in the refrigerator or freezer.

Potato starch flour: Made from potatoes, this fine white flour keeps well and is excellent for baking if sifted several times and used in recipes that include eggs. It can also be utilized as a thickener.

Rice Polish: Soft, fluffy, and cream-colored, this flour is made from the hulls of brown rice. Much like rice bran and high in nutritive value, it has a short shelf life. Buy it fresh and store in the refrigerator or freezer.

Sorghum flour: A fairly new product ground from specially bred sorghum grain, it is best used in combination with other gluten-free flours, stores well on the pantry shelf, and can be substituted for rice flour.

Soy flour: Smooth textured and nutty in flavor, its defatted type is lower in fat and will store longer. Soy flour should be stored in the refrigerator or freezer (due to its shorter shelf life), is best when used in combination with other gluten-free flours because of its strong flavor, and has a high nutritive content. If you are sensitive to soy, bean flour can be substituted for soy flour in most recipes.

Sweet rice flour: Called "sticky rice" and made from a glutinous rice, this is an excellent thickening agent, especially in sauces that are to be refrigerated or frozen. Not the same as plain white rice flour, it helps to bind ingredients together when baking.

Tapioca starch flour: A light tasteless flour that comes from the root of the cassava plant, it adds a "chew" factor to baked goods, is excellent for thickening soups, creams, gravies, puddings, and gravies. It can be stored on the pantry shelf for long periods of time.

Quinoa flour: Slightly bitter in flavor, this makes excellent biscuits and pancakes.

Whole bean flour or
Romano bean flour: Dark and strong in taste, these flours are milled from the Romano or cranberry bean. They are high in fiber, protein, and other nutrients. Products made with these flours are denser and require less for best results.

Other flour combinations include:

(1 cup = 1 cup wheat flour)

Both of these flour mixtures have a long shelf life and can be stored at room temperature.

This blend is also known as Bette Hagman's "Gluten-Free Gourmet Blend"* and is very popular. It is a heavy mix but will exchange well, cup for cup, with wheat flour when you are adapting recipes. Because of it's low protein content, the mix calls for adding extra protein and/or leavening, such as egg whites, dry milk powder, gelatin, or egg replacer.

Bette Hagman's Gluten-Free Gourmet Blend

2 cups white rice flour   1/3 cup tapioca flour
2/3 cup potato starch flour

This flour is available already mixed through Ener-g Foods at *www.ener-g.com*.

Bette Hagman's "Four Flour Blend"* also exchanges cup for cup with wheat flour. This mix does have enough protein so you should not have to add extra. The only other addition you would have to make when adapting your recipe is xanthan gum.

Gluten-free Substitutions*

Substitutions for 1 Tablespoon Wheat Flour

1/2 Tbs.	Cornstarch	7 mL
1/2 Tbs.	Potato starch or flour	7 mL
1/2 Tbs.	White rice flour	7 mL
1/2 Tbs.	Arrowroot starch	7 mL
2 tsp.	Quick-cooking tapioca	10 mL
2 tsp.	Tapioca Starch	10 mL
2 Tbs.	Uncooked rice	30 mL

Substitutions for 1 cup (240 ml) Wheat flour**

Mix:	2 cups	Brown rice flour	500 mL
	2 cups	Sweet rice flour	500 mL
	2 cups	Rice polish	500 mL

Store in an airtight container and use 7/8 cup (215 mL) of the mixture in place of 1 cup (240 mL) wheat flour.

Other Substitutions for 1 cup (240 mL) Wheat flour

5/8 cup		Potato starch flour	150 mL
7/8 cup		White or brown rice flour	215 mL
1 cup		Corn flour	240 mL
1 cup		Fine cornmeal	240 mL
3/4 cup		Coarse cornmeal	175 mL
	5/8 cup	White or brown rice flour	150 mL
Plus	1/3 cup	Potato starch flour	75 mL
	1 cup	Soy flour	240 mL
Plus	1/4 cup	Potato starch flour	50 mL
	3/4 cup	Rice flour	175 mL
Plus	1/4 cup	Cornstarch	50 mL
7/8 cup		Whole bean flour	215 mL

* ©2000, American Dietetic Association. "Manual of Clinical Dietetics, 6e." Used with permission.

** A combination of flours/starches gives a better gluten-free product.

Bette Hagman's Four Flour Blend

2/3 cup Garfava bean flour   1 cup cornstarch
1/3 cup sorghum flour   1 cup tapioca flour

This flour is also available already mixed through Authentic Foods and can be purchased at *www.glutenfree-supermarket.com.*

*Source: Used with permission from Bette Hagman, *The Gluten-Free Gourmet Living Well Without Wheat, Revised Edition*. (New York: Henry Holt and Company, LLC, 2000).

It is important to add either guar gum or xanthan gum to your gluten-free baked goods to compensate for the lack of gluten. This will add texture and affect the appearance of the overall food. When using xanthan or guar gum, the basic formula for breads is 3/4 teaspoon per cup of flour; for cakes 1/2 teaspoon per cup of flour, and for cookies 1/4 to 1/2 teaspoon per cup of flour.

Keep in mind that some gluten-free flours are very perishable. Store them in an airtight container in the freezer or refrigerator and label them with the date you made them so you can keep track of how long you have stored them.

When you are in need of a gluten-free baking powder try the following:

1/3 cup baking soda   2/3 cup arrowroot
2/3 cup cream of tartar   (or potato starch)

Mix well and store in an airtight container.
1 1/2 tsp. of this mixture = 1 tsp. of regular baking powder

Tips for the Gluten-free Baker and Cook

- Start with simple recipes until you have mastered the art of cooking with gluten-free flours and products.

- Modify your favorite recipes by substituting gluten-free flours and other ingredients. Try starting with recipes that already incorporate gluten-free flours.

- Most gluten-free flours *do not* substitute cup for cup with wheat flour, so use the previous chart to substitute the correct amounts.

- When you substitute gluten-free flour for wheat flour, you will usually get the best results with recipes that call for only a small amount of flour (less than 2 cups).

- Recipes that call for cake flour will do well when substituted with gluten-free flour.

- Use xanthan gum or guar gum in all of your yeast recipes to make the product springy.

- Gluten-free flours require using more leavening agents than with wheat flours. Add a little extra baking powder and/or baking soda to boost rising properties of your product.

- Baked goods turn out better when combinations of gluten-free flours are used. Brown or white rice flour plus potato starch flour and tapioca works well in breads. Potato starch flour plus cornstarch work well in pizza dough, and white rice flour plus tapioca works well for cakes.

- Put a pan of water in the oven when you are baking your product to help keep in the moisture.

- When using glass-baking dishes, reduce the oven temperature by 25 degrees.

- For extra flavor and moisture try adding nuts, fruits (such as applesauce or mashed banana), dried fruits (such as raisins), yogurt, or honey. Also try adding a little extra oil or shortening if you feel your recipes are too dry.

- Sift your flour and mixes before and after measuring them. This will help to improve texture.

- Add an extra egg or egg white for improved smoothness and crumb structure.

- Use Knox or any other unflavored gelatin in your baking recipes to help add moisture and help bind the ingredients. Before adding, mix the powder with half the water called for in the recipe.

- Beat gluten-free breads by hand with a wooden spoon or spatula. The batter is usually too thick for a whisk. This keeps the batter from being over-beaten and from becoming too fine and falling when baked.

- Using smaller pans will yeild a better product. Try using bun rings, muffin tins, bundt pans, and very small bread pans. If you can't find the right size or shape try using aluminum foil and folding it into the shape that you want.

- Use 1 1/2 tsp. cream of tartar and 1 tsp. baking soda for two loaves of bread. It will not interfere with the yeast and will help the bread to rise and help to keep it up during the baking process.

- When baking cookies, refrigerate the cookie sheet for half an hour before baking them to help keep the cookies from spreading too much.

- Refrigerate gluten-free dough for at least half an hour or better yet overnight to help soften the dough for a better textured product.

- Try replacing a small amount (about 1 Tbs.) of gluten-free flour with glutinous rice or sweet rice flour for baked goods such as brownies.

- Try substituting buttermilk for milk or water in gluten-free breads. This can result in a lighter and more finely textured product.

- Cornstarch and tapioca work the best for thickening foods such as sauces and gravies.

- To bind meat loaf or meatballs, try using plain popcorn that is blended into crumbs.

Some of the previous tips were adapted from *Gluten Free Diet: A Comprehensive Resource Guide, Revised Edition*, by Shelley Case B. Sc., RD (Case Nutrition Consulting, 2002).

Choosing a Bread Machine

Bread machines have become quite popular over the years, though not all machines are suited for making gluten-free breads. Some people prefer to use them whereas others prefer to make bread by hand. If you decide to invest in one, keep some of these important features in mind:

☐ Because gluten-free dough is heavier and harder to mix, choose a machine that has larger paddles.

☐ If the machine has an oblong, loaf-shaped pan, choose one that has two large paddles instead of one large paddle in the center. This will prevent the need to continually scrape the corners during the kneading process.

☐ Find a model that can be programmed for one rising cycle.

☐ Find a model that allows you to switch manually from knead to rise to bake, thus allowing you to manually control all the cycles.

☐ Gluten-free bread is usually made on the short or rapid cycle of the machine. Some of the machines will mix only once on this setting; others may mix twice. To get the best use out of your machine, you should be able to stop it at the dough stage and take the dough out so you can use it for other things besides bread.

☐ Find a model that has a cool-down cycle so the bread will not become soggy if it sits in the pan without being removed immediately.

☐ If you choose not to freeze bread, look for a model that offers a smaller bucket for a smaller size loaf.

There are many different types of bread machines on the market today. Talk to others who bake with them and ask for their recommendations.

Keep these tips in mind when baking bread with your bread machine:

☐ If there is dry flour sitting on the top of or in the corners of the dough, then it probably needs more liquid and/or better mixing. Add warm water (1 tsp. at a time), mixing after each addition, until the dough is smooth and less dry.

☐ If the batter is too thin (the consistency of cake batter) and has no defined lines on top, then it probably needs more dry ingredients. Add 1 Tbs. of rice flour at a time, stirring after each incorporation, until the dough is thicker and will pull away from the sides.

☐ Use flour and eggs that are at room temperature.

☐ Use warm ingredients (not hot) to help the bread to rise.

☐ Use milk and butter, instead of water and oil, to add moisture to the bread and create a chewy crust.

Preventing Cross Contamination

Not only is it important to make sure you check for gluten in the ingredients of the foods you eat, but it is also just as important to be aware of possible cross contamination with gluten-containing foods. This happens when a gluten-free product somehow comes into contact with something that contains gluten. At home, contamination can occur when your foods are prepared on common surfaces or when utensil or appliances are not cleaned thoroughly after use with a gluten-containing food. On an even larger scale, contamination can occur in manufacturing plants if separate machines are not used or if thorough cleaning does not take place between the production of batches. It is important to minimize cross contamination as much as possible. It doesn't take much for the intestinal villi of the person with celiac disease to become damaged with small amounts of gluten-containing foods. Following some simple steps can help reduce the chances for cross contamination.

- Implement a new "no double-dipping" rule in the household. Double-dipping is when a knife is dipped into a spreadable type condiment (such as peanut butter, jelly, mayonnaise, margarine), spread on the bread, and then dipped into the condiment again. The condiment becomes contaminated with the gluten-containing crumbs. Squeeze bottles make a good alternative if possible. You can also have the family use a spoon to get condiments out of the container and then spread it with a knife, stressing that they be careful not to touch the spoon to the bread. If other family members can't seem to stop double-dipping, buy separate condiments and label them as gluten-free and non-gluten-free. You can buy one large container of a product and than divide it into two smaller containers. Label each container so you know which is gluten-free. If the family uses up the non-gluten-free jar first and there is still quite a bit left in the gluten-free jar, give it to them to use up more quickly.

- Designate certain appliances for use only with gluten-free products. Toasters can be a big source of contamination because of the crumbs it can produce. Either designate a slot in the toaster that is only for gluten-free bread or buy a separate toaster for gluten-free products. Using a toaster oven that has a shelf that can be wiped clean after each use can also work.

- Make sure to wash utensils, cutting boards, other surfaces, pots, and pans thoroughly after each use. Also, wipe counters right before use, because wheat flours can stay airborne for many hours and contaminate exposed preparation surfaces and utensils.

- Store gluten-free products in separate labeled containers. You may even want to place gluten-free products in a separate cupboard and designated shelf in the refrigerator. You can use colored labels or other types of labels to help make sure everyone in the family as well as caregivers know which products are gluten-free.

- When preparing gluten-free and non-gluten-free foods at the same time (such as pasta), make sure you use separate utensils and food preparation tools. It may be easier to prepare one at a time.

- Purchase a separate set of utensils and other items needed for gluten-free cooking and baking. This includes buying separate paddles and bowls if you have a bread machine that is used for both regular and gluten-free breads.

- Tell babysitters or other caregivers who may be in the house how and why separate foods are needed. Stress the importance of not mixing foods, utensils, and/or appliances.

- When making any type of dip, put some aside for the person who is eating gluten-free if non-gluten-free food will be dipped into the main batch.

- Do not share nonstick and cast iron cookware with gluten-containing foods. They can be very porous. A better choice is stainless steel cookware.

- Use aluminum foil on baking sheets or pans that are also used for foods containing gluten.

- Purchase a separate colander for your gluten-free pastas. This is safer because it is quite hard to get colanders completely cleaned, even in the dishwasher.

- Avoid buying products such as flour from bulk bins. Scoops that have been used in bins with gluten-containing products could contaminate the gluten-free products.

- When eating at restaurants, be aware that French fries (even though they might be gluten-free) may have been fried in the same oil that battered gluten-containing foods have been fried in.

- When eating at restaurants specifically ask if the cook can clean the grill before preparing your foods and to keep your meal away from other meals that might contain gluten. You may want to call ahead to the restaurant to make sure it can handle your request.

- Be extra careful at buffet or family style restaurants because utensils being used in more than one serving pan can contaminate serving spoons.

- When questioning manufacturers about gluten-free foods, even if they state their food is gluten-free, make sure to ask if different machines are used for gluten versus gluten-free foods or if machines are cleaned in between production of batches.

Some tips adapted from *Gluten Free Diet: A Comprehensive Resource Guide, Revised Edition*, by Shelley Case, B. Sc., RD (Case Nutritional Consulting, 2002). *www.glutenfreediet.ca*

5 Preparing Everyday Gluten-free Meals

Planning Ahead

Meal planning for the gluten-free diet means one thing: planning ahead. There are many foods that are naturally gluten-free. This means there are many foods you don't have to give up. There are even more of your favorite foods (such as pasta, bread, and baked goods) that can be made from gluten-free grains and taste just like the foods you are used to. If you have a stocked kitchen and the foods that you need, you can make great easy meals and snacks at any time.

When preparing gluten-free meals for the person with celiac disease, make sure to avoid cross contamination by following some of the tips in Chapter 4. Start with safe food choices such as fresh meats, fresh fruits and vegetables, eggs, cheese, rice, potato products, corn, and soy. Avoid flours made from wheat, rye, barley, and any derivative of these flours. Avoid breads, rolls, croutons, bread crumbs, cakes, pies, cookies, muffins, noodles, crackers, and cracker crumbs made with gluten-containing flours. Avoid soups, sauces, and gravies as well as batters that may be thickened with these flours. To help you get started use some of the menu ideas in this chapter, but remember only to use this as a *starting point* to developing your own favorite meals and snacks. Eating a variety of foods is the best way to consume a variety of nutrients for good health.

The following is an excerpt from "The Newly-Diagnosed Celiac and DH'er: Step-By-Step: Beginning the Gluten-Free Lifestyle" *(www.houstonceliacs.org)* by Janet Y. Rinehart and Lynn Rainwater:

Meal Planning

☐ Plan meals before you get to the grocery store. The first couple of months will be frustrating when going grocery shopping because you are new at reading labels and, yes, gluten-free specialty products are more expensive. It's just a fact.

☐ To save time and trouble, plan on making as much of the meal gluten-free as possible. The person with celiac disease will appreciate not feeling different, and the cook will not have to make two meals. The "civilians" in the family can add gluten-containing bread or dessert items as they want.

☐ Start with simple meals, rather than combination dishes.

☐ Pay attention to all food sensitivities of your family.

☐ Make a rough draft of your meals for the next week, taking into consideration the family's schedule. Plan for the main entree, veggies, fruit, and salad. Plan one new, interesting gluten-free dessert each week.

☐ Use the CSA (Celiac Sprue Association) Commercial Product List to evaluate brand names of products (*www.csaceliacs.org*). Then make a brand-name grocery list based on the recipes you plan to use. Working on a weekly basis helps you eliminate extra trips to the grocery store, which will, in turn, reduce the frustration of looking at labels again and may save money.

☐ Be sure to plan for the family's snacks, both gluten-free and non-GF. When you have gluten-free items readily available (such as nuts, popcorn, fruit, and raw cut-up vegetables) you will be less tempted to "cheat" when you are starving.

☐ Try at least one new gluten-free recipe a week. Mark your cookbooks with comments, or develop a list of your favorites with the cookbook page noted. Include the family in meal-planning. What kind of meals do they like? Try to find good gluten-free substitutes.

☐ Make good use of your freezer. Freeze single portions of dinners to use as lunch items. Freeze dessert items for snacks.

☐ There are many companies that manufacture gluten-free specialty products. These products are more expensive than the comparable; that's just a fact. However, many of the mixes, frozen meals, and already-baked goods are quite good and make your life easier. See the CSA (Celiac Sprue Association) Products booklet for a listing of some of the specialty food manufacturers (*www.csaceliacs.org*). There are several online grocery stores with extensive gluten-free product lists. You may want to consult support group members to get their opinion of some of the products before you invest in a big order.

ALWAYS READ LABELS!!!

Start Your Day out Right: Breakfast Ideas

GF = Gluten-free

- GF cold cereal, sliced fresh fruit, fat-free milk, juice.

- GF frozen waffles or pancakes, sliced strawberries, syrup, fruit juice.

- Hard-boiled egg, home fried potatoes, GF toast, margarine, fat-free milk, fresh fruit.

- Hot cereal (cream of rice, cream of buckwheat) topped with raisins and cinnamon, fat-free milk, 1/2 of a grapefruit.

- Fruit smoothie: GF yogurt, skim milk, and fresh fruit blended together. (There are smoothie machines on the market today that make smoothie-making easy, and you can add just about anything you want to make a delicious and nutritious smoothie for any meal or snack.)

- GF bagel with peanut butter, GF yogurt mixed with blueberries, fruit juice.

- Breakfast sandwich: GF English muffin, scrambled egg, cheese, ham, and fruit juice.

- Hash browns cooked and mixed with scrambled eggs, onions, and bell peppers; and fruit juice or fresh fruit salad.

Time for a Lunch Break: Lunch Ideas

- Corn tortilla wrapped around GF tuna salad and GF cheese, fresh fruit salad.

- Homemade chili, GF corn chips, sour cream, tossed salad with GF salad dressing, grapes.

- Homemade egg salad on toasted GF bagel, fresh fruit, and GF yogurt.

- Whole potato, baked and topped with cheese, broccoli, and GF salsa; tossed salad and GF dressing; applesauce.

- GF English muffin topped with GF pizza sauce, mozzarella cheese, and any vegetable toppings you choose (just warm or broil in oven), tossed salad with GF dressing.

- Chef salad with vegetables, cheese, sunflower seeds, hard boiled egg, and grilled chicken breast (or your favorite meat), GF salad-dressing served with a GF bread stick that was brushed with margarine and garlic powder and heated in oven.

- Corn tortilla filled with chopped grilled chicken, GF cheddar cheese, GF salsa, diced tomatoes, and GF sour cream. Serve with fresh strawberries.

- GF rice noodle soup and grilled cheese and tomato sandwich made with GF bread.

- Chicken salad served on top of mixed greens and GF roll with margarine.

- Hummus (chickpeas, sesame seed oil, garlic) with GF crackers, fresh vegetables, and GF ranch dressing.

- GF hot dog on GF bun, GF baked beans, carrot sticks, and GF ranch dressing.

- Hamburger topped with grilled onions and GF cheese served on a GF bun served with GF tortilla chips and GF salsa.

- Cottage cheese served with fresh, sliced peaches.

- GF Pasta salad and fresh fruit.

Super Suppers: Dinner Ideas

- Barbecue pork or chicken using GF sauce, served with brown rice with toasted almonds and broccoli.

- Sweet and sour GF meatballs served over rice with a side of steamed vegetables.

- Grilled chicken breast topped with GF sharp cheddar cheese and GF salsa served with cooked brown rice mixed with GF salsa and steamed broccoli.

- Chicken quesadilla: grilled chicken and GF cheese between two corn tortillas; lightly brown on both sides in large fry pan sprayed with GF cooking spray. Top with GF salsa, GF sour cream, lettuce, and diced tomatoes.

- GF pasta mixed with ground beef, cooked zucchini, and GF spaghetti sauce, tossed salad with GF salad dressing, GF garlic bread.

- Pizza on GF crust or corn tortilla topped with your favorite meats, vegetables, and cheeses served with tossed salad and GF dressing.

- Grilled salmon, swordfish, or halibut drizzled with mixture of GF soy sauce, honey, ginger, and garlic powder served with red potatoes and fresh asparagus.

- Shish kebobs with your favorite meat and vegetables (such as steak, chicken, shrimp, bell peppers, onion, mushrooms, tomatoes, zucchini) served over brown rice.

- Steak, baked potato topped with margarine and GF salsa, tossed salad with GF dressing.

- Ground beef, GF taco seasoning, GF shredded cheddar cheese, chopped lettuce and tomatoes, black olives, GF salsa, and GF sour cream served in corn tortillas, corn taco shells, or over corn tortilla chips.

- Homemade meatloaf with garlic and cheese mashed potatoes (homemade mashed potatoes mixed with GF cheddar cheese and garlic powder to taste) and steamed green beans.

- Chili, GF corn bread, and tossed salad with GF dressing.

- Beef, chicken, shrimp, or tofu stir fry with vegetables and bean sprouts, served over brown rice.

Got the Munchies?: Snack Ideas*

- Corn chips.

- String cheese.

- Raisins or other GF dried fruit.

- Popcorn.

- Plain corn nuts.

- Hard boiled egg.

- Celery with cream cheese or peanut butter.

- Fresh vegetables and GF ranch salad dressing.

- Fresh fruit.

- GF bread with peanut butter.

- GF pudding.

- Jell-O made with fresh fruit.

- GF crackers and cheese.

- GF rice cakes.

- Applesauce sprinkled with cinnamon.

- Homemade trail mix: peanuts, M&Ms, raisins, chocolate chips.

- Apple with peanut butter.

- GF nuts.

- GF yogurt and fruit.

- Fruit smoothie (see page 84).

See Chapter 6 for recipes that will help with these menu ideas.

*Some meal ideas from *Gluten Free Diet: A Comprehensive Resource Guide, Revised Edition*, Shelley Case, B. Sc., RD (Case Nutritional Consulting, 2002). *www.glutenfreediet.ca*

Favorite Meals From the Experts

The following are meal ideas from people who have celiac disease who wanted to share some of their favorites. Thanks everyone!

(All oven temperatures are Fahrenheit.)

Regina Celano from Ronkonkoma, NY

Chili Potato

Microwave a baked potato. Open a can of Hormel Chili with beans (or any GF chili) and pour over potato, sprinkle with GF shredded cheddar cheese, and microwave again until cheese is melted.

Tex Mex Salad

Open a bag of salad from the grocery store, put some of the salad on your plate (I use a pasta dish). Microwave GF Chili and pour over the salad, top with GF shredded cheddar cheese and GF sour cream. Dip GF tortilla chips into the mixture. (Would be great with GF salsa on top, too!)

Pizza

Take a frozen Chebe Bread Pizza Crust out of the freezer. (When you make them, make a few and freeze the rest for future use). Top with GF pizza sauce and GF shredded cheese and any other GF topping of your choice: onion, mushrooms, broccoli, chicken (whatever you prefer). Pop in the oven and dinner is served!

Chicken Salad Platter

Open a can of chicken and make chicken salad, scoop out a healthy portion on top of a bowl of salad, from the bag. Microwave some cheesy Parmesan bread sticks you made from your Chebe Bread Mix and have in your freezer.

Zesty Mac and Cheese

Make a box of GF macaroni and cheese, mix in a can of GF chili and heat through. Serve with carrot and celery sticks on the side.

Tacos

Ground beef or chicken tacos are great. Just make sure your taco mix/seasoning; shredded cheddar cheese and sour cream are all GF. Serve with lettuce, tomato, black olives, GF sour cream, and GF salsa.

Burgers

Buy ground beef to make your own hamburger patties. Make extra and freeze them so you can take out one or two and grill them when needed. When you make Kinnik-Kwik Bread Buns, make a few extra and freeze them, too.

Stacy LaRoche from New York, NY

This is very fast if you have a pressure cooker and use real risotto, which I prefer. If you don't have a pressure cooker, use instant rice, as directed. A pressure cooker will cook up real risotto in about the same amount of time as it takes to make instant rice and has a great deal more flavor.

Italian Bacon and Tomato Risotto

Cook sliced bacon (about 1/2 lb) and 1 chopped onion in a skillet. Drain.

Stir in a few handfuls of halved cherry tomatoes, 14 ounces GF chicken broth, 1/2 cup of milk (or milk substitute if you can't tolerate milk), 1 tsp. dried parsley (or fresh parsley to taste), and 2 cups of instant rice.

Bring to a boil over medium heat. Simmer for 5 minutes over low heat. Add GF grated cheese to taste (you can use parmesan, Romano, etc.). Let stand 5 minutes. Serve topped with GF grated cheese.

Jessica Duvall from Williamsburg, KS

Chicken Broccoli Stir Fry

Cut 1 lb. of boneless, skinless chicken breast into chunks or strips and cook in small amount of oil until cooked through.

Add 1/3 cup GF soy sauce, garlic to taste, and 1 1/2 cups water; bring to a boil.

Stir in 2 cups broccoli and 2 cups instant brown rice. Cover and cook over low heat for approximately 5 minutes or until rice is done.

Kit Kellison from Chesapeake, VA

Crunchy Chicken

Prepare a shallow baking dish with GF cooking spray, and preheat oven to 400 degrees. Mix 2 Tbs. milk and 1 beaten egg. Dunk 6 pieces chicken in egg mixture, salt and pepper both sides, roll in 1 cup crushed GF cornflake crumbs. Salt and pepper again, place on baking dish, and dot with butter.

Bake for 1 hour or until chicken is cooked through. Easy, and one of the best GF breading recipes there is. The chicken comes out moist, tender, crispy, and delicious!

Lila Brendel from Bismarck, ND

Pasta Dinners

Brown ground beef, add various GF pastas, and use your favorite seasonings, tomatoes, GF cheese, vegetables, or anything else you want to add. Great variety and takes 20 minutes to prepare a meal.

Fajitas

Corn tortilla with melted cheese and your favorite meat, mushroom, onion, bell pepper (any color), GF salsa or (be creative), in the center.

Great Summer Potatoes

Use whatever vegetables you prefer and amount you need. Try potatoes (cut into cubes), zucchini, carrots, green beans, green/red/yellow peppers, onion, butter, seasoning salt, and pepper.

Put ingredients in a 9 x 13 pan. Cover with about 2 Tbs. butter and add about 1/2 cup water. Cover with foil and bake at 400 degrees for 30 minutes or until vegetables are tender (or put mixture in foil and grill).

Creamed Potatoes and Vegetables

Five to 6 cut up potatoes, 1 bag frozen vegetables (carrots, broccoli and cauliflower), 1 pint whipping cream, salt, and pepper. Place potatoes in large frying pan. Add salt, pepper and 1/2 cup water, cook until almost tender, stirring frequently. Add vegetables and cream, and cook until cream bubbles and vegetables are hot.

More easy favorites:

☐ Sausage and hash browns.

☐ Seasoned and grilled chicken breasts with rice, GF pasta, or potato.

☐ Sweet and sour chicken or shrimp served over rice.

Marcy Thorner from New Market, MD

Keep things simple when preparing family meals: A grilled meat, rice or potatoes prepared your favorite way, steamed or stir-fried veggies, and salad makes a simple, enjoyable meal that the whole family can enjoy and is healthy for all. A GF child who can eat whatever is on the table will feel less isolated.

Joyce Etheridge from Avon, IN

Sloppy Joes

I have a very simple recipe for Sloppy Joes that is a quick meal. I make it two different ways covering our food allergies.

Regular Gluten-free/corn-free Sloppy Joes:

1 lb. regular ground beef
3–4 Tbs. regular brown sugar
1/2 onion chopped
Muir Glen Organic Ketchup, as much as needed

Sloppy Joes for Candida/corn-free:

1 lb. ground Buffalo meat
2 Tbs. Turbino or substitute brown sugar
1/2 onion chopped
Muir Glen Organic Ketchup, as much as needed

We spoon the mixture on buns that are gluten-free, yeast-free/gluten-free, and regular (depending on the person). Serve with salad (lettuce with carrots, tomatoes, cucumbers, peppers) and vegetables or potatoes.

*Tip: I make the regular one normally with a 3-lb. package of ground beef and then freeze little packages of them for a quick meal later.

Ashley Cooper from Urbandale, IA

Quick and Delicious Pizza!

1 Kinnikinnick pizza crust
Virgin olive oil with garlic
1 cup low-fat mozzarella shredded cheese
Fresh tomato slices
Cut up mushrooms

Spread the olive oil on the pizza crust. Add your tomato slices and mushrooms. Cover with mozzarella cheese. Bake at 350 degrees for 15 minutes.

Rolf Meyersohn from New York City, NY

Polenta and Risotto

I use a microwave oven to make polenta (based on cornmeal) as well as risotto (based on Arborio rice), without having to stir endlessly. Barbara Kafka's *Microwave Gourmet* has excellent recipes for these dishes as well as many others.

Chicken Stock

I make chicken stock every month or so, from bones collected and frozen from our roast chicken. A stockpot is essential. Homemade chicken stock works well, especially in risotto, where salt-free (not to mention gluten-free) stock is needed.

Cover chicken carcass and bones with water; add a carrot, celery stalk, an onion, a bay leaf, and peppercorns. Simmer for 1 1/2 hours (90 minutes).

Socca

"Every morning the streets of Nice are full of men carrying large round trays of socca on their heads (wrapped with handkerchiefs) to the marketplaces and shouting 'tout caud'."

—*The Cuisine of the Sun* by Mireille Johnston

Mix 2/3 cup chickpea flour, 3 tablespoons olive oil, 1/4 tsp. salt, 1 cup water, ground pepper; rest 1 hour or more at room temp or in refrigerator.

Preheat oven to 400 degrees. Oil a round shallow [nonstick] pan and pour on batter, about 1/8 inch thick. Put under a moderate broiler as close to flame as possible. After 5 minutes sprinkle a little olive oil on top and broil for 5–10 minutes more until it is crisp and golden with the consistency of a thick crepe. Slide onto serving plate and cut into 2-inch wedges.

Barbara Westmoreland from Hampstead, NH

Breakfast Sandwich

Pull two pieces of frozen GF bread out of the freezer, give them a quick zap, and toast them. Fry an egg with melted cheese thrown on after flipping. Put it all together to make the most delicious, nutritious sandwich. You can also make the sandwich on a corn taco shell or wrap it in a corn tortilla and also add GF bacon, ham, or Canadian bacon. Eat half a can of fruit cocktail for dessert.

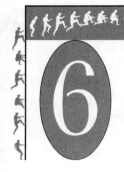

Delightful Gluten-free Recipes

There are all kinds of great gluten-free recipes out there to try. Look into cookbooks and Websites that can help (see Chapter 9). The following recipes come from all types of sources and can help you get started on your way to delicious gluten-free cooking.

Wake up Your Taste Buds: Breakfast Recipes
Ham and Cheese Omelet with Fresh Basil
Serve with hash browns, orange slices, and tomato juice
From Kit Kellison, Chesapeake, VA

1/4 cup chopped onion
1 oz. shredded sharp white
cheddar *or* Asiago (or your
favorite full-flavored) cheese
2 thin slices GF deli ham, rolled
and sliced into thin strips

3 eggs, well beaten
3-4 leaves chopped fresh basil
1 Tbs. butter or olive oil
Salt and pepper to taste

In an omelet pan (GF Teflon or stainless steel), sauté onions on medium heat until they begin to brown and release a sweet aroma. Add the ham and cook until slightly brown. Add the basil and eggs, mixing in the cheese before the egg sets too much.

This will make it a bit more quiche-like. Lift the mixture up off the pan occasionally to let the uncooked egg run to the bottom. When the bottom is cooked well, flip the mixture over to cook the other side. It is important to use enough oil and not to let the pan get too hot to do this properly and to keep the egg from sticking to the pan. Fold the omelet on the plate while sprinkling some extra cheese in the middle and on top, if desired. Cover with a pot lid for five minutes to let the cheese melt and the flavors blend a bit before serving.

Prep time: 5 minutes   Cooking time: 15 minutes

Pancakes and Blueberry Sauce
Serve with syrup and fruit juice
With permission from Allan Gardyne, Best Gluten-Free Recipes
http://members.ozemail.com.au/~coeliac/det.html

Pancakes:

1 cup brown rice flour	1 1/4 cups water
1 cup white rice flour	2 eggs

Blend everything except the eggs in a food processor. Allow the mixture to stand for at least two hours. Add the eggs and beat. Brush a frying pan with oil. Pour in some of the mixture. Cover with a lid and cook on medium-low heat about 5 minutes. Turn with a spatula and cook the other side. Repeat.

Sauce:

1 oz. butter	1 Tbs. brown sugar
1/4 cup blueberry jam	1/3 cup chicken stock (can
2 tsp. arrowroot	use gluten-free stock cubes)
1/3 cup red wine	

Melt butter and jam in a saucepan over low heat. Add stock, red wine, sugar, and arrowroot. Keeping it on a low heat, stir until the sauce thickens. Serve over pancakes.

Cheesy Potato and Ham Casserole

With permission from Allan Gardyne, Best Gluten-Free Recipes
http://members.ozemail.com.au/ ~ coeliac/det.html

3 medium potatoes,
   peeled and thinly sliced
1 onion, sliced
2 hard-boiled eggs, chopped
3/4 cup grated GF cheese
1/4 cup cooked GF ham,
   chopped

1/2 cup milk
2 Tbs. GF chutney
1/4 tsp. paprika
Freshly ground black pepper
Herb salt

Grease an oven-safe dish. Add half the potato and onion slices. Sprinkle with salt and pepper. Spread the cheese, ham, chutney, and eggs over the potato slices. Pour the milk over mixture. Use the remaining potato and onion slices to make another layer. Add the milk and sprinkle with paprika.

Bake in 360-degree oven for about 30 minutes. The potatoes should be tender.

Microwave version: Microwave for 15 to 20 minutes.

Delicious Dining: Lunch and Dinner Recipes

Fast Beef Stroganoff

Serve over brown rice with steamed spinach
With permission from Allan Gardyne, Best Gluten-Free Recipes
http://members.ozemail.com.au/ ~ coeliac/det.html

1/2 lb. ground beef
1 packet GF onion soup mix
3 cups GF rice noodles
1/2 tsp. ground ginger

3 1/2 cups hot water
1 can sliced mushrooms
1 cup cream
Maize corn flour or cornstarch

Microwave meat on high for 5 minutes. Add packet of soup, noodles, ginger, hot water. Cook 12 minutes. Add mushrooms and cream and thicken with maize corn flour. Microwave for another minute.

Carol Fenster's Pizza Crust & Pizza Sauce
Top with mozzarella cheese and vegetables.
Serve with salad and GF dressing
With permission from Carol Fenster, Ph.D., Savory Palate, Inc.,
www.savorypalate.com

Pizza Sauce:

1 can (8 oz.) tomato sauce	1/2 tsp. fennel seeds
1/2 tsp. dried oregano leaves	1/4 tsp. garlic powder
1/2 tsp. dried basil leaves	2 tsp. sugar
1/2 tsp. crushed dried rosemary	1/2 tsp. salt
	Toppings of your choice

Combine all ingredients in small saucepan and bring to boil over medium heat. Reduce heat to low and simmer for 15 minutes, while pizza crust is being assembled. Makes about 1 cup.

Pizza Crust:

1 Tbs. dry yeast	1 tsp. Italian herb seasoning
2/3 cup brown rice flour or garbanzo/fava bean flour*	2/3 cup warm milk (110°) or non-dairy liquid
1/2 cup + 2 Tbs. tapioca flour	1/2 tsp. sugar or honey
2 tsp. xanthan gum*	1 tsp. olive oil
1/2 tsp. salt	1 tsp. cider vinegar
1 tsp. unflavored gelatin powder (Knox)	Extra rice flour for sprinkling

*Available at health-food stores by Authentic Foods, Bob's Red Mill, Gluten-free Pantry, Ener-G Foods, and Miss Roben's.

Preheat oven to 425 degrees. In medium mixer bowl using regular beaters (not dough hooks), blend the yeast, flours, xanthan gum, salt, gelatin powder, and Italian seasoning on low speed. Add warm milk, sugar, oil, and vinegar. Beat on high speed for 2 minutes. (If the mixer bounces around the bowl, the dough is too stiff. Add water if necessary, 1 tablespoon at a time, until dough does not resist beaters.) The dough will resemble soft bread dough. (You may also mix in bread machine on dough setting.) Put mixture on lightly greased 12-inch pizza pan. Liberally sprinkle rice flour onto dough, then press dough into pan, continuing to sprinkle dough with flour to prevent sticking to your hands. Make edges thicker to hold the toppings. Bake pizza crust for 10 minutes. Remove from oven. Top pizza crust with sauce and your preferred toppings. Bake for another 20–25 minutes or until top is nicely browned. Serves 6 (1 slice per serving).

Spaghetti Pie
Serve with tossed salad and GF dressing
With permission from Connie Sarros, author of Wheat-free Gluten-free Cookbook for Kids and Busy Adults, www.homestead.com/gfkids/gf.html

1 Tbs. olive oil	1/2 tsp. basil
4 cups cooked, GF spaghetti (about 1/2 lb. uncooked)	3/4 tsp. oregano
	1/4 tsp. garlic powder
2 cups GF spaghetti sauce	1 Tbs. parsley flakes
1/2 cup GF grated Parmesan cheese	1/2 cup GF grated mozzarella cheese
1/4 tsp. red pepper flakes	

Preheat oven to 350 degrees. Pour oil into a 9-inch pie plate. Use a pastry brush to spread it on the bottom and sides of the pan. Put spaghetti into a large bowl. Use a clean pair of scissors to cut it into smaller pieces. Pour the spaghetti sauce over the spaghetti. Sprinkle the Parmesan cheese, red pepper flakes, basil, oregano, garlic powder, and parsley over the spaghetti. Stir spaghetti with a fork to mix thoroughly. Pour spaghetti into pie plate. With the back of a spoon, pat it down. Sprinkle top with mozzarella cheese.

Bake for 30 minutes. Make sure an adult removes the dish from the oven. Cut the "pie" into wedges to serve. Serves 6.

Note: When cooking spaghetti, cook it al dente (just barely tender).

Crock Pot Pork Chops

Serve with GF au gratin potatoes and steamed cauliflower
With permission from Connie Sarros, author of Wheat-free
Gluten-free Cookbook for Kids and Busy Adults,
www.homestead.com/gfkids/gf.html

1 lb. pork chops	1/2 cup GF Italian dressing
1/2 tsp. garlic powder	1 small bottle GF barbecue
3 Tbs. GF soy sauce	sauce

Wash pork chops under cold running water. Pat dry with paper towels. Sprinkle garlic powder on both sides of chops. Place chops in a large self-seal plastic bag. Pour the soy sauce and the Italian dressing into bag. Seal bag securely. Push bag around gently to distribute the dressing between the chops. Refrigerate bag several hours.

Remove pork chops from the marinade and place in a crock pot. Pour the barbecue sauce over the chops, lifting the chops with a fork to distribute the sauce evenly. Cover crock pot and cook on low for 8 hours. Serves 6.

Super Easy Chicken

With permission from Connie Sarros, author of Wheat-free
Gluten-free Cookbook for Kids and Busy Adults,
www.homestead.com/gfkids/gf.html

1 Tbs. light brown sugar	2 Tbs. GF ketchup
3/4 cup GF salsa	4 boneless skinless chicken
	breast halves

Preheat oven to 400 degrees. In a small bowl, stir together the brown sugar, salsa, and ketchup. Lay the chicken pieces in an 8 x 12 baking pan that has been sprayed with gluten-free, nonstick spray. Spoon the salsa mixture over the chicken pieces. Let the chicken marinate at room temperature for 20 minutes.

Bake for 40 minutes or until the chicken is cooked through. Have an adult help you remove the hot pan from the oven. Serves 4.

Almost Cheeseburger

With permission from Connie Sarros, author of Wheat-free
Gluten-free Cookbook for Kids and Busy Adults,
http://www.homestead.com/gfkids/gf.html

1/2 lb. lean ground beef	1/4 cup milk
1 tsp. dried minced onion flakes	2 Tbs. GF ketchup
1 lb. GF processed cheese, cut into cubes	2 Tbs. GF mustard

Have an adult help you brown the beef and onion flakes in a skillet that has been sprayed with a gluten-free nonstick spray, breaking up the meat with a fork as it cooks. Stir in the cheese, milk, ketchup, and mustard; stir until the cheese has melted.

Note: Use as a dip with crackers, as a "cheeseburger" with GF bread "fingers" as dippers, or as a main meal by serving it over boiled, gluten-free elbow macaroni.

Yields 4 cups. Serving size: 1/2 cup.

Mexican Lasagna

From Clare Popowich, Belchertown, MA

1 lb. ground beef or turkey	1 can GF tomato sauce or salsa
1 pkg. GF taco seasoning mix	1 pkg. corn tortillas
1 can GF refried beans (can be fat-free)	1 pkg. shredded cheddar (or your favorite) cheese

Prepare beef and taco seasoning mix according to package directions. Mix refried beans and tomato sauce or salsa, reserving about 1/2 cup of sauce or salsa for the top. Spread a little bean mixture into casserole to keep tortillas from sticking. Layer tortillas, bean mixture, and cheese, ending with tortillas. Spread with reserved tomato sauce/salsa and sprinkle with cheese. Bake 350 degrees until bubbly. This can be prepared ahead of time and reheats well. Serve with taco condiments. If you prefer your dishes cheesier or saucier, increase ingredients accordingly.

The following three recipes are copyrighted by Clan Thompson and reprinted with permission. To learn more about celiac disease, you can visit Clan Thompson online at *www.clanthompson.com*.

Meatloaf

1 cup GF bread crumbs
1 onion, chopped and
   lightly fried
1 egg, slightly beaten
1 Tbs. GF soy sauce
3/4 tsp. dry mustard

1/4 tsp. garlic powder
1/4 tsp. salt
1/4 tsp. black pepper
1/4 cup milk
1 lb. ground beef

Mix all the ingredients together in a large bowl. Place into a greased pan. Bake in a preheated 350-degree oven for about one hour. If you want leftovers for meatloaf sandwiches, you may want to double the amounts!

Chicken Pot Pie

www.clanthompson.com

Crust: Use the "My Favorite Pie Crust" recipe (see page 103).

Filling:

6 Tbs. butter
6 Tbs. cornstarch
3 cups milk
1 tsp. salt
1/4 tsp. black pepper

1/4 tsp. crushed garlic
16-oz. package frozen vegetables
4–6 chicken thighs, cooked, or
   an equivalent amount of
   breast or leg meat

Melt butter in a heavy-bottomed saucepan over low heat. Slowly add cornstarch and blend well. Gradually add milk, blending well. Continue to stir as the sauce thickens. Bring to a boil and reduce heat, stirring for another 2–3 minutes. Remove from heat. Add salt, black pepper, and crushed garlic. Add one 14–16 oz. package of frozen vegetables. I prefer the Bird's Eye combination that includes pea pods, carrots, peas, and baby corn. Add the chicken.

Place the bottom crust in a 8- or 9-inch pie pan. Fill pan with the chicken, vegetables, and sauce. Make a lattice crust to cover the pie. Cook at 350 degrees for 45 minutes or until done.

My Favorite Pie Crust

www.clanthompson.com

2/3 cup cornstarch	1 Tbs. white sugar
2/3 cup soy flour	2/3 cup Crisco
2/3 cup tapioca flour	1 egg
1 tsp. baking powder	5 Tbs. cold water
1 tsp. xanthan gum	Cornstarch for rolling
1 tsp. salt	

Put the flour, baking powder, xanthan gum, salt, and sugar into a medium bowl. Cut in the Crisco until you have small pieces the size of lima beans. Mix the egg and the 5 tablespoons cold water in a separate cup. Add 5 tablespoons of this mixture to the flour and stir well. If necessary, add more liquid until the dough forms into a ball. Refrigerate at least an hour to chill.

Divide the dough in half. Roll the first half out onto a board dusted with cornstarch. Transfer to a pie tin. If the crust breaks, just piece it together in the pie tin and press the dough back together. Fill the crust with appropriate filling. Use the remainder of the dough to cut strips for a lattice crust. Cook at 350 degrees or as recipe for filling directs. Makes one two-crust pie.

Quick Chili

With permission from www.Planetceliac.com—*the gluten-free place to be!*

1 lb. ground beef	1 Tbs. chili powder
1/3 cup milk	1 8-oz. can GF tomato sauce
1 medium onion, chopped	1 16-oz. can kidney beans

Sauté beef and onion in a large skillet. Drain excess oil. Add tomato sauce, milk, chili powder, and kidney beans. Simmer 45 minutes to 1 hour.

Gouda Burger

Serve with GF tortilla chips and GF salsa

Recipe provided with permission from www.Glutenfreeda.com.

1/2 lb. ground beef
1 shallot, minced
2 tsp. Worcestershire sauce
Salt and freshly ground black
  pepper
1 large garlic clove,
  minced and divided

2 Shiitake mushrooms, sliced
1 Tbs. olive oil, divided
2 1/4-inch slices of a beefsteak
  tomato
1/2 cup mixed salad greens
1/4 cup sliced Gouda cheese
Herbed mayonnaise (see
  recipe on page 105)

In a large bowl, combine the ground beef, shallot, 1/2 of the minced garlic, and Worcestershire sauce. Form hamburger mixture into 2 1/2-inch thick patties. Season patties with salt and freshly ground black pepper. Set aside.

In a small skillet, heat 1/2 Tbs. of olive oil over medium heat. Add the remaining garlic, and sauté for 30 seconds. Add the mushrooms and sauté for 3–4 minutes or until the mushrooms are tender and lightly browned. Remove from heat and set aside. Heat the remaining 1/2 Tbs. of olive oil in a large skillet over medium-high heat. Add the hamburger patties and cook for 4 minutes per side, or until nicely browned on both sides and cooked through.

To assemble the burger, place the beefsteak tomato slice in the center of a plate. Top the tomato with a hamburger patty and spread 1 heaping Tbs. of the herbed mayonnaise over the top of the burger. Top with 1/2 the cheese and 1/2 the sautéed mushrooms. Garnish the top of the burger with mixed greens. Repeat assembly with remaining burger. Serve immediately. Makes 2 servings.

Herbed Mayonnaise:

1/4 cup mayonnaise
1 Tbs. fresh basil, chopped

2 tsp. Italian parsley, chopped

Combine in a small bowl.

Baked Chicken Supreme

With permission from www.Planetceliac.com—*the gluten-free place to be!*

1 frying chicken, skinned
  (about 1 1/2 lbs.)
1 green pepper, cut into strips
1 clove garlic, pressed
1/4 cup scallions, chopped
1 cup GF chicken stock

1 tsp. tarragon
1/2 cup margarine or butter
2 tomatoes, cut into wedges
1 tsp. paprika
1 tsp. salt

In 1/4 cup of margarine, brown chicken on both sides with garlic and paprika. Remove from pan. Add remaining margarine and sauté mushrooms, onions, and green pepper. Return chicken to pan. Add chicken stock, tarragon, tomatoes, and salt. Simmer for 1 hour or until chicken is tender. Serve over rice.

Herbed Crusted Chicken w/Poblano Cream Sauce

With permission; recipe provided by www.Glutenfreeda.com.

4 chicken quarters
  (leg & thigh attached)
2 Tbs. cumin seeds
1/2 tsp. chipotle powder or
  chili powder

2 Tbs. roasted garlic, chopped
2 tsp. salt
2 tsp. peppercorns, crushed
2 Tbs. olive oil

Preheat oven to 375 degrees. In a small bowl, combine cumin seeds, chipotle powder, garlic, salt, crushed peppercorns, and olive oil. Rub generously over washed and dried chicken pieces. Place chicken in a baking dish and bake for 1 hour and 20 minutes (or 80 minutes). After 45 minutes, remove chicken from oven and baste with pan juices and continue basting every 15 minutes until done.

Poblano cream sauce:

2 Tbs. olive oil
1 poblano chile, chopped
3/4 cup onion, chopped
4 cloves garlic, minced
3/4 cup cilantro, chopped

1/4 cup whipping cream
1/2 cup crème fraiche,
    or GF sour cream
Salt and pepper to taste

Heat oil in a heavy saucepan over medium heat. Add chile and onion and sauté until onion is just translucent. Add garlic and sauté for 1 more minute. Add remaining ingredients and simmer for 2 minutes until sauce is blended and slightly thickened. Season with salt and pepper. Transfer sauce to a food processor and process until smooth.

Remove chicken from oven and spoon a layer of sauce on tops of chicken quarters. Return to oven for 10 minutes. Serve immediately. Makes 4 servings.

Shrimp and Fish Tacos
Serve with GF Mexican rice and GF mayonnaise
Recipe provided with permission from www.Glutenfreeda.com.

> *Tip: This recipe takes a bit of prep but is well
> worth the effort. Instead of broiling the fish and
> shrimp, you can grill them if you prefer.

For the tacos:

6 Tbs. ground dried New
    Mexico or California chilies,
    or 1–2 tsp. red pepper flakes
3 Tbs. salad oil
1/2 tsp. pepper
1/2 tsp. salt
1/2 tsp. garlic powder
1/2 tsp. cayenne
1/2 tsp. ground cumin
2 whole cloves

1 dried bay leaf, broken into
    pieces
3/4 lb. boned, fresh skinned
    firm-flesh fish such as
    halibut or mahi-mahi
1/2 lb. medium size prawns,
    peeled and deveined
1/4 cabbage, sliced thin
12 GF corn tortillas

In a large bowl, mix ground dried chilies, oil, pepper, 1/2 tsp. salt, garlic powder, cayenne, cumin, cloves, and bay leaf. Rinse fish and shrimp; pat dry. Add to bowl and turn to coat with marinade; cover and chill at least 1 hour or up to 1 day, mixing several times.

For the Pico de Gallo:

2 cups diced tomatoes
1/2 cup finely diced onion
2 Tbs. minced jalapeño chili
1/4 cup minced fresh cilantro

2 Tbs. lime juice
1 garlic clove, minced
Salt to taste

In a bowl, combine all ingredients. Salt to taste.

For the Cilantro-Jalapeño Mayonnaise:

1 3/4 cup GF mayonnaise
 (see recipe on page 108)
2 Tbs. water
2 Tbs. cider vinegar
1 jalapeño chili

1 garlic clove
1/2 cup lightly packed cilantro
1/4 teaspoon pepper
Salt to taste

In a blender or food processor, combine all ingredients. Whirl until smooth. Add salt to taste.

Heat tortillas one at a time over medium high heat in a heavy skillet. Keep warm by wrapping in foil.

Lift fish from marinade and arrange pieces in a single layer in a 9 x 13-inch pan. Discard marinade. Broil fish 4–5 inches from heat until opaque but still moist-looking in center of thickest part (cut to test), about 5 minutes for 1/2 inch thick pieces. With a slotted spatula, transfer fish to towels to blot oil, then set on a platter. Cut fish along the grain into 1/2-inch slices and shrimp into 1/2-inch pieces; season to taste with salt.

To assemble tacos:

Spread a layer of cilantro-jalapeño mayonnaise on a heated tortilla, top with fish and shrimp mixture, cabbage, and pico de gallo. Enjoy!

GF Mayonnaise

With Permission; recipe provided by
http://www.Glutenfreeda.com.

Tips: For perfect results every time, use a food processor with an attachment that allows liquid to be added in a very small stream. Fill with oil and process while oil is added very slowly.

1 whole egg	1/2 tsp. salt
1 tsp. GF stone-ground mustard	Fresh ground white pepper
	Dash of cayenne
1 Tbs. lemon juice	1 cup vegetable oil

Add all the ingredients to a food processor or blender except the oil. Blend briefly. With the motor running add the oil in a slow, thin, steady stream. After the mayonnaise is made, correct the seasoning to taste. Makes 4 servings.

Lighten It Up: Soups and Salads
Tex-Mex Pasta Salad

With permission from The Gluten-free Pantry, *an online book by Beth Hillson, Gluten-free Pantry staff, and their customers.* (www.glutenfree.com)

1 10-oz. package gluten-free fusilli or elbow rice pasta	1 cup cubed cooked chicken, optional
1 14.5-oz. can black beans, rinsed and drained	1 cup medium salsa (check labels)
1 cup frozen corn kernels, thawed	1/2 cup plain yogurt or low-fat sour cream (check labels)
1 red bell pepper, seeded and chopped	3 Tbs. GF mayonnaise
3 green onions, chopped	2 tsp. ground cumin
	Salt and pepper to taste

Cook pasta, drain, and rinse in cold water. Combine drained pasta, black beans, corn, pepper, green onions, and chicken, if used. In a separate bowl, combine salsa, yogurt or sour cream, mayonnaise, cumin, and salt and pepper. Pour over pasta mixture and stir to blend. Refrigerate until ready to serve. Serves 8.

Lentil Soup

The following recipe is copyrighted by Clan Thompson and reprinted with permission. To learn more about celiac disease, you can visit Clan Thompson online at *www.clanthompson.com.*

1 1/2 Tbs. oil
1 large onion
1 clove garlic
1/3 cup brown rice
2 cups dried lentils, washed and picked over
2 quarts cold water
1 hambone with meat
2 potatoes, peeled and cut
2 sliced carrots
1 large rib of celery, chopped
1/4 cup (scant) celery leaves chopped
1 cup of tomato juice
1 tsp. dried basil
2 Tbs. chopped fresh parsley or 2 tsp. dried parsley
1/2 cup dry white wine
Salt and pepper to taste

Cook the onion, garlic, and brown rice in a pot with the oil for 5 minutes over low heat. Add lentils, 2 quarts cold water, and the hambone. Bring to a boil and cook 1 hour. Add potatoes, carrots, celery rib and leaves, tomato juice, basil, parsley, salt, and pepper. Cook until vegetables are tender for 30 to 60 minutes. Cut meat off bone and remove bone. Stir in 1/2 cup of dry white wine and serve. Replenish water while cooking as needed. Serves 10–12.

Betsy's Creamy Potato Cauliflower Soup

Serve with tossed salad and GF dressing and Yummy
Breadstick (see page 114)
With permission from The Gluten-free Pantry,
www.glutenfree.com.

1 1/2 cups potatoes peeled
   and diced
2 small celery sticks, diced
1 small onion, minced

1 1/2 cups water
1 1/2 cups cauliflower in small
   florets, steamed for 5 minutes
1 tsp. salt

Cook everything but the cauliflower until tender. Mash (do not drain). Add cauliflower.

White sauce:

2 Tbs. butter
   substitute

1 1/2 cups milk or milk
2 Tbs. cornstarch

Bring white sauce ingredients to a boil and stir continuously until mixture thickens. Fold into soup. Garnish with parsley and serve. Serves 4.

Jazz It up: Sauces

Aunt Catey Sauce

From Tim Coda, Salt Lake City, UT

This recipe is named after my great aunt Catey. She always seemed to have this on hand on the farm in Illinois.

3 Tbs. butter
1 Tbs. peanut oil (or substitute
   more butter)
3/4 cup onion, diced finely

3–5 cloves garlic, minced,
   depending on your own
   tastes (I use 5 or 6)

Sauté previous ingredients and add:

3 cups milk (whole, 2-percent, 1-percent, or skim)
1–1 1/2 cups Velveeta cheese, cubed in 1/2-inch cubes
Pinch salt and pepper
1 tsp. basil
1/4 cup white wine (optional)
2–3 Tbs. corn starch dissolved in equal amounts cold water

In saucepan, sauté garlic and onions in butter and oil. Add milk, wine, and seasonings and heat on low for 5 to 10 minutes. Slowly add cheese, stirring constantly as it **will** scorch to the bottom of the pan until just about to boil. When just beginning to boil, thicken with cornstarch mixture.

Serve over vegetables, seafood, GF pasta, whatever you want. My father used to say, "This would even make shoe laces edible."

Be the Life of the Party: Appetizers and Party Foods

Chebe Bread Piggies-in-a-Blanket

From Regina Celano, Ronkonkoma, NY

1 cup shredded cheese (your choice)
2 eggs
2 Tbs. oil
1/3 cup water
20 GF cocktail weiners or GF sausages

Using a bread dough mixer, or with a spoon blend cheese, eggs, oil, and water. Mix well with hands for 5 minutes or until very smooth and well-blended. (Add a little water if too dry; add Chebe mix or food starch if too sticky.) Roll into 20 balls and flatten each one. Place a cocktail wiener or sausage on each piece of dough and roll them up. Place on non-greased baking sheet and bake until golden brown.

Salsa-Cheese Dip/ White Sauce
From Kit Kellison, Chesapeake, VA

2 Tbs. butter
1 Tbs. potato flour
1 cup milk

4 ounces shredded Kraft
mild cheddar cheese
1 Tbs. GF salsa

Make a roux by melting butter over medium heat and stirring in the potato flour until it starts to bubble. Turn up heat a bit and slowly add milk until it thins the roux into a set pudding-type texture. Thin a little more, then stir for a couple of minutes to allow the flour to cook and to make sure the mixture doesn't get too thick. Add more milk as needed, and watch your heat. If you have gotten this far, you have just made a white sauce that can be adapted to make any other milk gravy, cream sauce, or soup you would like.

When the sauce is at milk-gravy consistency, stir in 1 ounce of the cheese at a time, stirring in between until it is all blended and melted. At this point you might want to taste the mixture to see if it is cheesy enough. You may add more cheese if you prefer, incorporating it in slowly, mixing all the while. When the mixture is smooth, add the salsa, which will bring the color up and add a nice tang. Serve with heated tortilla chips.

Layered Taco Dip
From Regina Celano, Ronkonkoma, NY

1 8-oz. package of softened
GF cream cheese
1 8-oz. bag of GF shredded
cheddar cheese

1 can of Hormel chili with
beans
1 large bag of GF tortilla chips

In a microwave-safe 8 x 8 pan spread the softened cream cheese, top with the contents of the can of chili, and pour the bag of shredded cheddar over the chili. Microwave until the cheese gets bubbly.

Open the bag of GF tortilla chips, dip, and enjoy!

Chicken Wings
From Lila Brendel from Bismarck, ND

4 lbs. chicken wings or
    drumsticks
1 cup GF soy sauce
1 cup water
1/4 cup oil

1/2 cup pineapple juice
1 tsp. ginger
1 tsp. garlic
1 cup sugar

Mix ingredients and marinate chicken overnight. Bake on cookie sheet at 350 degrees for 1 1/2 hours (or 90 minutes). (Can keep warm in crockpot.)

Everyone's Favorites: Desserts and Breads
Our Best Bread
Reprinted with permission from www.Planetceliac.com—*the gluten-free place to be!*

1 stick margarine
3 large or 3 1/2 small,
    very ripe bananas
1/2 cup butter, softened
2 cup rice flour (*or* prepared
    GF baking mix)

1 cup sugar
1 cup pecans, finely
    chopped or ground
2 eggs
2 tsp. GF baking powder
1 tsp. GF vanilla

In a large bowl, cream butter with sugar. Beat in eggs, vanilla, and bananas. In another bowl, stir and mix together flour and baking powder. Combine and beat with banana mixture until dry ingredients are moist. Stir in pecans. Turn batter into 5 x 9 loaf pan. Bake at 325 degrees for one hour and 20 minutes (or 80 minutes) or until toothpick comes clean out of center. Do not underbake. Yields one loaf of 10 large slices. Toasts very well with pecans added as finely ground flour.

Yummy Breadsticks

Reprinted with permission from The Gluten-free Pantry,
www.glutenfree.com.

Combine:

1 bag *Bagel Mix*	1 Tbs. GF yeast
1 tsp. salt	1–2 tsp. each, dry basil and
3 Tbs. grated Parmesan cheese	oregano

Mix together:

1 egg plus 1 egg white, lightly beaten	2 Tbs. honey
	1 tsp. cider vinegar
2 Tbs. olive oil	1 egg yolk plus 1 Tbs. warm
1 cup warm water	water to brush breadsticks

Preheat oven to 425 degrees. Beat liquids into dry ingredients using a heavy-duty mixer. Beat for two to three minutes or until mixture is smooth. Roll into 10, 9-inch lengths between layers of oiled plastic wrap. Transfer to breadstick pan or baking sheets. Cover with oiled plastic wrap and let rise 30–40 minutes. Brush with beaten egg yolk mixture and sprinkle with coarse salt. Bake 16–18 minutes. Cool slightly before serving.

Banana Nut Bread

With permission from www.Planetceliac.com—*the gluten-free place to be!*

1 cup rice flour	3 tsp. GF baking powder
3 eggs	1/2 cup corn oil
1 cup potato starch	3 large or 4 small bananas, mashed
1/2 cup sugar	
1/2 cup soy flour	2 Tbs. water
1/2 tsp. salt	1/2 cup chopped nuts

Mix flours, starch, and baking powder. Blend together eggs, sugar, salt, oil, and water. Blend in the mashed bananas. Stir in the dry ingredients. Add the nuts. Pour into an 8 1/2 x 4 loaf pan. Bake at 350 degrees for an hour.

Harvest Pumpkin Bread/Cupcakes/Muffins
From Connie Rieper of Fayetteville, AR

1 cup brown sugar
1/3 cup butter, softened
 or cooking oil
1/2 tsp. GF vanilla extract
2 eggs
1 can pumpkin
1/4 cup milk (use soy milk
 or juice if you have other
 food intolerances)

1 cup flour mix (I use white
 rice, potato starch,
 tapioca, xanthan gum)
1/2 tsp. salt
1/2 tsp. ginger
1/2 tsp. nutmeg
1/4 tsp. ground clove
 (don't overuse the cloves!!)
2 tsp. cinnamon
1 1/2 tsp. baking powder

Preheat oven to 250–275 degrees. Grease pans. In large bowl, cream butter and sugar with mixer. Add vanilla, eggs, pumpkin, and milk in order. Mix well.

Mix all dry ingredients together. Add to the large bowl. Blend wet and dry ingredients together. Add walnuts and raisins. Pour into cupcake, muffin, or bread pans. Bake small cupcakes/muffins for 20 minutes, larger cupcakes/muffins for 30 minutes, and bread for 40 minutes. Check them with wood skewers to see if the center is cooked (no dough on skewer). Cooking times may vary with different ovens. When cooled, frost the cupcakes with GF frosting.

GF Poori (fried bread from India)
From Connie Rieper, Fayetteville, Arkansas

1 cup GF flour mix
 (or white rice flour)
1/2 tsp. salt

2 Tbs. oil
7 to 10 Tbs. milk or water

Pour flour in bowl. Add salt and mix. Dribble oil over the top and rub it into the flour with your fingers. Slowly (1 Tbs. at a time) add milk, or water, to form a medium-soft ball. Knead for 10 minutes, or until smooth. (It should have consistency of new Play-dough: no dry cracks, but not soggy or slimey.) Form big ball, cover with oil, let rest. Divide dough into 12 balls. Take one, roll it out into about a 2- or 3-inch round (cut a Zip-loc baggie into two plastic squares and roll the dough in between—easy to lift dough off of—or hand-flatten in two hands).

Use a deep, frying pan, or wok, over medium high heat. When oil is very hot, lay poori carefully on surface of oil without letting it fold up. It should sizzle immediately (if it doesn't, heat oil more). Spoon hot oil over poori or dunk it under with a spoon with quick strokes. It should puff up in seconds. Turn poori over and cook for a few seconds. Remove with slotted spoon and place on paper towels. Serve immediately.

5-inch, flattened rounds will make crispy crackers, but will not puff up.

Lime Meringue Pie

The following recipe is copyrighted by Clan Thompson and reprinted with permission. To learn more about celiac disease, you can visit Clan Thompson online at *www.clanthompson.com*.

1 1/2 cups sugar
5 Tbs. cornstarch
1/8 tsp. salt
1 1/2 cups hot water
2 egg yolks, slightly beaten
Rind of 1/2 lime, grated
2 Tbs. butter

1/3 cup lime juice
1 8- or 9-inch pastry shell
  (pre-baked and gluten-free)
2 egg whites
1 tsp. lime juice
6 Tbs. sugar

Mix 1 1/2 cups of sugar, cornstarch, and salt in a saucepan. Blend in the hot water, gradually. Bring to a boil over high heat, stirring constantly. Reduce heat to medium. Cook and stir for 6 more minutes. Remove from heat. Stir a small amount of the hot mixture into the egg yolks and then add to the rest of the hot mixture. Bring to a boil over high heat, stirring constantly.

Reduce heat to low and cook and stir constantly for 4 more minutes. Remove from heat. Add lime peel and butter. Stir in 1/3 cup lime juice. Cover surface with clear plastic wrap and cool for 10 minutes. Pour into your favorite pre-baked gluten-free pastry shell. Cool to room temperature. To make meringue: Beat egg whites with 1 tsp. lime juice until soft peaks form. Gradually add 6 Tbs. sugar, beating until stiff peaks are formed. Spread meringue over the pie, making sure to seal to edges of pastry. Bake in a moderate oven (350 degrees) for 12–15 minutes or until the meringue is golden. Cool thoroughly before serving.

Buttermilk Brownies
From Jan Hammer, Fargo, ND

1/2 cup oil	2 eggs
1/2 cup buttermilk	2 cups sugar
1/2 cup margarine	2 1/4 cup flour mix (see below)
1 tsp. baking soda	4 Tbs. cocoa
1 cup cold water	

Bring water, margarine, and oil to a boil. Add baking soda to buttermilk. Pour over dry ingredients. Beat until creamy. Add buttermilk, soda, and eggs. Beat well. Bake in jelly roll pan (15 x 10) for 18 minutes at 400 degrees.

Dry Flour Mix:

2 cups brown rice flour	1 1/3 cup tapioca starch or flour
2 cups white rice flour	1/2 cup rice bran or rice polish
1 1/2 cup sweet rice flour	2 tsp. xanthan gum
2/3 cup cornstarch	

Sift all ingredients three or four times and store in canister. Use 1 cup of this mixture when recipe calls for 1 cup wheat flour. Works very well in cookies, bars, cakes—even rolled out sugar cookies.

Jelly Roll

From Jean Wright, Allegany, NY

1 cup GF flour mixture
  (see below)
1 tsp. baking powder
1/4 tsp. salt

3 large eggs (3/4 cup)
1 cup sugar
1/3 cup water
1 tsp. vanilla

Heat oven to 375 degrees. Grease a jelly roll pan (15 1/2 x 10 1/2 x 1) and line bottom with greased parchment paper or greased aluminum foil.

Blend flour, baking powder, and salt; set aside. Beat eggs in small mixing bowl until very thick and a light lemon color. (It takes a while!) Pour beaten eggs into large bowl. Gradually beat in sugar. Blend in water and vanilla, on low speed. Slowly mix in dry ingredients (low speed) until batter is smooth. Pour into pan. Bake 12 to 15 minutes. Loosen edges and immediately turn upside down on a towel sprinkled with confectioners sugar. Remove paper. Trim stiff edges. While hot, roll cake and towel starting with the narrow end. Cool on wire rack. Unroll cake, remove towel. Spread with soft (not syrupy) jelly or filling of your choice. Roll again. Sprinkle with confectioner's sugar. Cut in 1-inch slices. (You can cut it into 4 pieces widthwise and stack with filling (such as fresh strawberries) and top with whipped cream. If you want a chocolate roll just add 1/4 cocoa to dry ingredients.

You can fill with a clear orange or lemon filling or pudding!! It's soft and moist and flexible. Serve to anyone!!! They'll never know the difference!!!

GF Flour Mixture

2 cups GF garbanzo and
  fava flour
1 cup GF Sorghum flour
3 cups cornstarch

3 cups tapioca flour
2 slightly rounded tsp.
  xanthan gum

(Makes 9 cups. Keep refrigerated.)

Banana Bread or Muffins
From Jean Wright, Allegany, NY

3 over-ripe bananas, mashed
2 Tbs. butter, soft
1 cup sugar
1 egg
2 Tbs. buttermilk or "sour milk"*
1 tsp. baking soda

1/2 tsp. GF baking powder
1/2 tsp. regular or sea salt
2 cups flour (use GF mixture with 2 tsp. xanthan gum)
1/2 cup finely chopped walnuts (optional)
1/2 cup raisins (optional)

Preheat oven to 350 degrees. Grease and flour (with GF flour) loaf pan. Mix ingredients thoroughly. Pour into prepared loaf pan. Bake at 350 degrees for 1 hour. (For muffins (12) bake 25 minutes.)

*To make sour milk: Place at least 2 Tbs. milk in a dish and add a few drops of cider vinegar. Let sit 5 minutes until it curdles.

GF Orange Cookies
From Barbara Emch, Hubbard, OH

Preheat oven to 375 degrees.
Grate the rind from 5 oranges and squeeze the juice; mix together and set aside.

In medium bowl, wisk:

3 cups Bette Hagman's GF mix (see page 71)
1 tsp. xanthan gum

1 tsp. baking soda
2 tsp. GF baking powder

In a large bowl, cream:

1 1/4 cups sugar
1 cup shortening

3 eggs
1/4 cup applesauce

Add 1 cup of juice and rind to creamed mixture. Next, add the dry ingredients to the creamed ingredients and mix well. Drop teaspoonfuls 2 inches apart onto greased baking sheet and bake for 10–15 minutes. Frost with GF orange frosting.

Peanut Butter Christmas Balls*

From Teresa A. Van Nuland, Kenosha, WI

Tip: Crush cereal in a baggie to save on clean-up.

2 cups crushed cereal crumbs	1 tsp. vanilla
2 sticks margarine	5 Tbs. butterscotch chips
1/2 cup chunky peanut butter	5 Tbs. chocolate chips
2/3 cup well packed coconut	1/6 stick paraffin (wax found
3 cups powdered sugar	in grocery canning section)

Cream the margarine and peanut butter together. Next add powdered sugar gradually while mixing at low speed to avoid dust. Add coconut, cereal crumbs, and vanilla. Mix well and form into 1 1/4-inch sized balls by hand. Set balls aside.

Melt butterscotch and chocolate chips with paraffin in the microwave. (If this mixture cools, you may need to re-melt for use.) Dip balls to coat, then remove to cool on waxed paper. Makes approx. 40 balls.

*For Gluten-free adaptation, I use EnvironKidz brand "Gorilla Munch," Imperial margarine, Skippy/Jif PB, Baker's flaked coconut, Crystal powdered sugar, and Authentic Foods' brand Premium Vanilla Powder (reduce amount to 1/4 tsp. GF vanilla powder). For butterscotch and chocolate chips, I use Baker's/Hershey brand.

Thin Mint Cookies

(Tastes just like the Girl Scouts version.)
From Teresa A. Van Nuland, Kenosha, WI

40 unflavored round crackers	10 drops GF mint or
1/2 cup chocolate chips (use	peppermint extract
semi-sweet for slightly less	1/6 stick paraffin (wax found
carbs; use milk chocolate	in grocery canning section)
type for sweeter version)	

Melt chocolate chips and paraffin together in microwave, stirring occasionally to blend. Add drops of mint extract. Stir. Dip cracker into melted chocolate (using small tongs or fingers to coat). It may be necessary to reheat chocolate/paraffin mixture periodically as it begins to harden. Remove coated cracker and place on wax paper for drying. Store in refrigerator to prevent melting or store at room temperature if desired.

For GF brands, use Bi-Aglut snack crackers, Hershey or Baker's chocolate chips, and McCormick's brand of mint extract.

German Chocolate Cake
Recipe provided with permission from by
www.Glutenfreeda.com

Makes one 3-layer cake

Tip: Use the Gluten-Free Pantry's Country French Bread Mix as a straight substitution for flour.

2 1/4 cups GF flour
1 tsp. baking soda
1/2 tsp. salt
4 ounces semi-sweet
GF chocolate, chopped
1/2 cup boiling water
1 cup crème fraiche

1 tsp. vanilla
1 stick unsalted butter,
at room temperature
1/2 cup vegetable oil
1 3/4 cups sugar
5 large eggs

Preheat oven to 350 degrees. Grease and flour three 9-inch cake pans and line the bottoms with parchment paper.

In a medium bowl, sift together, flour, baking soda, and salt. Set aside. In a small bowl combine chocolate and boiling water and stir until chocolate is melted. Set aside. In a small bowl add 1 cup crème fraiche and vanilla. Set aside.

In a large bowl, beat 1 stick butter and oil on high until lighter in color and texture. Beat in sugar slowly. Beat in 5 egg yolks, one at a time. Add the chocolate and beat just until combined.

Alternately, add and beat on low speed, the flour mixture and the crème fraiche.

In a separate bowl, beat the egg whites until soft peaks form. Fold egg white mixture into the batter. Stir gently until combined and pour evenly into the cake pans. Bake for 30 minutes or until an inserted toothpick comes out clean. Let cakes cool on a rack.

For frosting:

1 cup sugar
1 cup crème fraiche
1 stick unsalted butter,
  cut into small pieces
3 large egg yolks
1 1/3 cups unsweetened
  coconut
1 1/3 cups pecans, chopped

Combine sugar, crème fraiche, butter, and egg yolks in a small saucepan and bring to a boil. Reduce the heat to low and cook for 1–2 minutes, stirring constantly. Remove from heat and stir in coconut and pecans. Let cool.

Remove one cake from the pan and place on a cake platter, right side up. With a sharp knife, cut the crown of the cake so it is flat. Top with 1/3 frosting; do not frost the sides of the cake. Repeat with remaining layers.

Ginger Bread People

From Bonnie J. Kruszka, author of Eating Gluten-Free with Emily, *(Xlibris Publishing, 2003) Newbury, OH*

1/2 cup shortening
2 1/2 cups Bette's Gourmet
  Four Flour Blend
  (see page 73)
1/2 cup sugar
1/2 cup molasses
1 egg
1 Tbs. vinegar
1 tsp. GF baking powder
1 tsp. ground ginger
1/2 tsp. baking soda
1/2 tsp. cinnamon
1/2 tsp. ground cloves

In mixing bowl beat shortening with an electric mixer on medium speed for 30 seconds. Add about half of the flour, the sugar, molasses, egg, vinegar, baking powder, ginger, baking soda, cinnamon, and cloves. Beat till combined. Beat in remaining GF flour. Cover and chill for 3 hours or till easy to handle.

Divide the chilled dough in half. On a lightly GF floured surface, roll half of the dough at a time 1/8-inch thick. Cut desired shapes with a 2 1/2 inch cookie cutter. Place 1 inch apart on a greased cookie sheet. Bake in a 375-degree oven for 5 to 6 minutes or until edges are lightly brown. Cool on the cookie sheet for about 1 minute. Remove and cool on wire rack. Makes about 36 cookies.

Chocolate Buttermilk Cake
From Marybeth Doyle, Kirtland Hills, OH

3/4 cup oil	2 cups fern soya powder
2 cups sugar	1/2 cup potato starch flour
2 tsp. vanilla	2 tsp. GF baking powder
4 eggs	1 tsp. baking soda
3–4 1-ounce squares baking chocolate	1 1/2 sticks margarine or butter, melted
1/2 tsp. xanthan gum	1 cup milk

Melt the chocolate and let cool. Cream oil, sugar, and vanilla. Add margarine or butter, beat, and then add eggs and beat well. Add the melted chocolate and mix. In a separate bowl, mix flours, xanthan gum, baking powder and backing soda. Add the dry ingredients, alternating with the milk, to the chocolate mixture. Blend well. Pour into greased (use Pam non-stick cooking spray) 11 x 8 cake pan. Bake at 350 degrees until a knife comes out clean.

Buttermilk frosting:

Cream together 1/2 cup real butter with 1/2 cup butter flavored Crisco (or regular). Then add 1 teaspoon vanilla and blend well. Add 1 cup at a time powdered sugar (4 cups total) alternating with 1 Tbs. milk (3–4 Tbs. total). Blend well and frost the cooled cake.

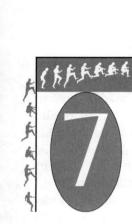

Gluten-free for All Occasions

Special Occasion Challenges

Special occasions are a part of everyone's life, whether you have celiac disease or not. Special occasions can include anything from parties to weddings to traveling to eating in restaurants. Many of these events involve eating food outside of the home. They can present new challenges for those on a gluten-free diet. The most important factor is to be prepared for whatever occasion you are about to encounter. Use the knowledge and skills you have learned and follow some of the helpful tips and information in this chapter. Keep in mind that no matter what the event is, the actual *special occasion* is what you are celebrating and is of greater importance than the food being served.

Party On

Parties come in all forms: dinner parties, birthday parties, Superbowl parties, holiday parties, office parties…. Who doesn't like a good party? The key is to be prepared. One tip is to fill up before you go. It is not a good idea for anyone to get to a party completely famished but, for the person on a gluten-free diet, it is an especially bad idea. Eat before leaving the house in case you are headed to a party where there may be limited gluten-free food choices. You can also call the host ahead of time to discuss what will be on the menu. Graciously ask if he or she can put a bowl of salad aside for you before adding croutons and/or salad dressing as well as a plain piece of meat, fish, or chicken before marinade, sauce, or breading is added. Offer to bring a dish or an appetizer so that you know for sure there will be something there that you can eat. Don't be afraid to ask questions when you eat at a party. Politely ask, "Oh, this looks delicious. What is in it?" And be careful of those utensils that get used for more than one dish or appetizer.

There are all types of great foods that you can serve or bring with you to parties. Adapt some of your favorite party recipes into gluten-free recipes. Good choices include GF birthday cake or other desserts, deviled eggs, GF tortilla chips and GF salsa, sweet and sour GF meatballs, fresh veggie tray with dip, fresh shrimp, hummus, assorted nuts, stuffed mushrooms, or barbecued chicken wings. Use your imagination! (See Chapter 6 for some great recipes!) At the buffet or appetizer table, seek out the fresh vegetables, fresh fruit, and cheese platters. These are usually the safest to eat.

Traveling Tips

Traveling can involve airplanes, trains, boats, or car trips. No matter what your means of transportation be sure to plan ahead here, too. If you are going to fly and your trip is long enough that you will be eating airline food, call the airline at least 24 hours in advance and request a gluten-free meal. There are a number of airlines that offer gluten-free meals.

The following airlines have been known to accommodate passengers that request gluten-free meals:

- Delta.
- American.
- Continental.
- Northwest.

- Air Canada.
- Lufthansa.
- British Air.
- Swissair.

- Virgin Atlantic.
- Air New Zealand.
- Qantas.

This is not an all-inclusive list, so be sure to call the airline you are taking to request information. If you have any doubts about the food that is going to be served, bring your own. Even though many airlines now serve gluten-free meals, their understanding of the gluten-free meal may not be up to par. If you order a special meal from the airline and there are breads, muffins, or cookies that have no wrapper, be careful because you won't be able to verify the ingredients. It is best to pack a few snacks to take with you in case your meal isn't quite what you expected.

If you are planning a cruise, compare different cruise lines and find out which ones might be more accommodating to your special dietary needs. Keep a few snacks in your room to eat throughout the day or take with you when you leave the boat for a full-day excursion. Most cruise lines will be accommodating to your dietary needs. Ask about bringing your own mixes for the chef to make up during your stay.

When planning for a car trip, pack a cooler to make sure you have plenty of food for the length of your trip. Pack crackers and cheese, peanut butter, GF granola bars, fresh fruit, fresh veggies, GF cookies, GF candy, or nuts. Don't forget to pack plenty of water, too!

When traveling out of the United States double-check the label and ingredient lists on foods that are labeled "gluten-free." Some countries are different in their labeling laws, so be sure you are not being served a product made with wheat starch. In many foreign countries products that are labeled gluten-free may contain up to .3 percent protein (which may possibly be gluten) and wheat starch is used in their baked goods. Corn flour can be modified food starch on many foreign labels, which means it can contain corn, wheat, or other flour. You can bring some of your own foods on your travel outside the United States but you may need to have a letter signed by your physician stating it is for medical purposes so that it will not be confiscated.

Research your destination and try to get recommendations about gluten-free friendly restaurants and hotels from local support groups or online message boards. People who live in the area or who have traveled there before can be a big help.

Dining Out

Dining out can be very frustrating for someone with celiac disease. All those choices on the menu that you cannot order.... Just as with diabetics, people with other food allergies or who are watching their weight must make special choices the person on a gluten-free diet must learn to make special choices that do not contain gluten. It is easy to avoid the obvious rolls, pasta, casserole dishes, and breaded meats, but you must look deeper. Has the meat been marinated in some type of sauce before it was cooked? Is the meat floured before it is grilled or broiled? Is the soy sauce made from wheat or soy? Is the rice steamed in water or some type of broth? Were there croutons in the salad that were simply picked out because you ordered it without? What are the ingredients in the salad dressing? It is important to ask questions. Don't be embarrassed to ask the server or even ask to speak to the chef. It is your health and you are paying for your meal! Many celiac organizations now offer "restaurant cards" that gives the chef or cook a simple explanation of your special dietary needs.

The sample Restaurant Card on page 129 is available at *www.glutenfree.com/celiac.htm*.

Restaurant Card

Use this card as a tool to help explain the gluten-free diet to your server and chef upon arrival at a restaurant in advance of your visit.

Guidelines for Preparing a Gluten-Free Restaurant Meal

I have a severe reaction to gluten and thank you for preparing a meal that I can safely eat. I appreciate your effort—plain and simple food is just fine.

I cannot digest the gluten in wheat, rye, oats, or barley. Even a crumb or speck of flour made from those grains will make me ill. Please be careful not to make my food in pans that have flour or crumbs on them from other food preparation. Please do not use oil that was previously used for frying breaded foods.

I cannot have bread, breadcrumbs, flour, whole wheat flour, semolina, soy sauce, rye breadcrumbs and flour, barley malt, pearl barley, orzo, oats, oat flour or oatmeal, starch (unless it's from corn, tapioca, or potato), modified food starch, hydrolyzed vegetable or plant protein, cakes, cookies, buns or rolls, and sauces made from canned or powdered stocks.

Please do not put croutons on or near my salad or breadcrumbs or toast on my food. Please do not put cookies in or near my dessert. I must also avoid low fat mayonnaise, yogurt, marinated foods, and foods covered in barbecue sauce (unless the ingredients are known). I cannot eat foods covered in most barbecue sauces and gravies.

Thank you for your help!

Using a card may help you to feel more comfortable when communicating with the restaurant staff. Make up your own card that you can carry in your purse or wallet for easy access or purchase one at Living Without *(www.livingwithout.com/ Diningcards.htm)*. You can also contact your local celiac organization or national organizations about these cards.

Before you dine out carefully choose the restaurant you are going to visit. Choose a restaurant with a large menu selection or restaurants with ethnic foods that are more likely to be gluten-free, such as Mexican, Thai, or Japanese. Avoid buffet-type places where you will not be able to easily find out what is in the foods and how they were prepared. Avoid French and Italian restaurants, where it may be difficult to find a dish that is gluten-free.

Most restaurants (even fast food ones) will offer some type of meal that is gluten-free. Remember everything you have learned about eating gluten-free and verify any questionable ingredients with the staff. If the waitstaff cannot help, ask to speak to the chef. Make sure you not only ask about specific ingredients but about food preparation procedures in the kitchen.

Here are some tips to follow when dining out:

- The chef and waitstaff may not be as knowledgeable as you about gluten-free diets, so be specific when asking about certain dishes.

- Explain to the staff that you have a serious food allergy and that their help is greatly appreciated. Be polite and descriptive about your dilemma, not demanding or difficult.

- Choose restaurants that have foods that are made to order and menu choices that are simple.

- Call the restaurant and talk to the manager or chef ahead of time to make sure they can accommodate your needs.

- Explain cross contamination and that your meal needs to be prepared using a separate pan and separate, clean utensils. Some restaurants will surprise you and be very helpful.

- Opt for a baked potato as a side dish instead of rice, which is often cooked in chicken stock or bouillon. Stay away from potato dishes that contain additional ingredients or potatoes that are fried (the same oil may be used for other batter-fried foods).

- Order menu items that are simple such as grilled chicken or broiled fish and ask them to top with fresh lemon, olive oil, or fresh herbs. Make sure it is not floured first.

- Begin with something basic such as plain meats, poultry, or fish instead of having the chef take away things that may be forbidden.

- Make sure that your salad does not contain croutons and did not come in contact with them.

- Bring your own salad dressing so you don't have to worry about checking the ingredients of the restaurants brands.

- Ask servers not to place garnishes on your dish in case they are not gluten-free.

- When ordering hamburgers, make sure they are 100-percent beef and have no fillers and that the hamburgers buns are not toasted on the same grill surfaces where the burgers were cooked.

- Take a look at the appetizer list. There is nothing wrong with potato skins topped with cheese and bacon bits or shrimp cocktail as a meal. Be careful of potato skins and nacho chips that are fried with gluten containing foods. Ask that your skins be baked instead of fried.

- If you feel comfortable, bring your own crackers, bread, or nachos.

Terms to Know When Eating Out		
Avoid	**Ask about**	**Order**
Au gratin	Soup	Fresh
Bisque	Stew	Grilled
Breaded	Dressing	Steamed
Coated	Fried food	Broiled
Casserole	Imitation	Poached
Creamed	Marinated	Roasted
Croutons	Sauce	Pan seared
Processed	Sautéed	
Roux	Soufflé	
Stuffing	Stir-fry	

Restaurants to Visit

Many restaurants are beginning to acknowledge gluten-free foods and dishes, so don't be afraid to eat out. Find specific restaurants in your area that you can trust will give you choices and serve you a safe gluten-free meal.

A few restaurant chains that do serve gluten-free foods include:

McDonald's

McDonald's has a corporate dietitian on staff and she has devised a gluten-free menu sheet for customers. The list basically includes McDonald's core items and not promotional, regional, or test items. The list is updated on a regular basis so always check back regularly. You can visit the Website at *www.mcdonalds.com* or call 1(800) 244–6227 to request a nutrition facts brochure. As always keep cross contamination issues in mind.

Some of the foods included on the list are:

- Beverages: coffee, hot chocolate, milk, orange juice, soft drinks.
- Chocolate, Strawberry and Vanilla Triple Thick Shake.
- Beef patty (no bun).
- Canadian bacon.
- Cheese.
- French fries (be sure that the store does not fry anything but fries in the same fryer).
- Fruit & yogurt parfait (no granola).
- Grilled chicken breast (no bun).
- Hash browns.
- Ham.
- Sausage.
- Scrambled egg.
- Chef and Garden McSalad Shaker.
- Dressings: Caesar, Fat-Free Herb Vinaigrette, Ranch, Red French Reduced-Calorie, Thousand Island.
- Ice cream sundaes, including nuts.

Taco Bell

Taco Bell has stated that because wheat is a part of so many of its recipes, many items served at Taco Bell restaurants are not suitable for gluten-free diets. However, there are a few items you can safely order:

- Pintos and cheese.
- Cheese sauce.
- Guacamole.
- Hot and mild sauce.
- Fiesta salsa.
- Sour cream.
- Seasoned rice.
- Jalapeno peppers.
- Three cheese blend.

Taco Bell has stated that its nacho chips, even though they do not contain wheat, are now fried at each store and are fried in the same fryer in which wheat-containing items are prepared. You can contact Taco Bell at 1(800) tacobell or visit the Website at *www.tacobell.com*.

Wendy's

The following items are gluten-free:

- Chili.
- Potato with chili and cheese.
- Grilled chicken salad.
- Taco salad.
- Fries.
- Frosty.

You can request additional information from Wendy's about the menu at:

Consumers Relations Department
Wendy's International, Inc., Dublin, OH 43017
(614) 764–6800
www.wendys.com

Arby's

Arby's is currently working with its vendors and suppliers to gather information necessary to compose a list of gluten-free products for its customers. It plans to have this information available on its Website in the near future. At this time Arby's does **not** use separate fryers for gluten and gluten-free items. At this time the only products specified by its suppliers to be gluten-free are:

- Arby's Roast beef.
- Arby's Horsey Sauce.
- Arby's Sauce.

You can learn more by visiting the Website *www.arbys.com* or calling 1(800) 487–2729.

Dairy Queen (DQ)

Dairy Queen lists gluten-free foods on its Website at: *www.dairyqueen.com*. The following items are listed as gluten-free:

- Vanilla and chocolate soft serve.
- Misty Slush.

Its supplier of manufactured novelties also states the following are gluten-free:

- Cherry-Lime and Lemon Freez'r.
- DQ Fudge Bar.
- DQ Vanilla Orange Bar.
- DQ Vanilla Fudge Bar.
- DQ Raspberry Vanilla Bar.
- StarKiss Bars.

Dairy Queen also notes to check all of this information with your local restaurant. The corporate number is 1(952) 830–0200.

Boston Market

Gluten-free menu items:

- Butternut squash.
- Chicken, rotisserie.
- Whole kernel corn.
- Cranberry relish.
- Creamed spinach.
- Fruit salad.
- Plain grilled chicken breast.
- Green beans.
- Hot cinnamon apples.
- Jumpin' Juice Squares.
- Mashed potatoes.
- New potatoes (garlic and dill).
- Turkey breast, rotisserie.
- Vegetables, steamed with glaze.

Boston Market Corporation
14103 Denver West Parkway
Golden, CO 80401
1(800) 365–7000
www.bostonmarket.com

Subway

Subway provides information on many allergens in its foods including wheat and gluten. The following foods are wheat- and gluten-free:

Salads:

Veggie Delight, Turkey Breast, Turkey Breast & Ham, Ham, Roast Beef, Subway Club, Tuna, Italian BMT, Cold Cut Trio, Subway Melt.

Meats:

Turkey breast, ham, roast beef, Subway Club meats, plain chicken strips, Seafood and Crab, tuna, Italian BMT meats, Cold Cut Trio meats.

All of Subway's condiments and fixings are gluten-free.

The list is updated regularly. You can check the Website at *www.subway.com* or call 1(800) 888–4848.

Outback Steakhouse

Outback Steakhouse is very accommodating to gluten-free patrons. It has a menu online that can be printed out to let you know which menu items are gluten-free. At this time the gluten-free items include:

- Grilled Shrimp on the Barbie.
- Queensland Salad.
- Brisbane Caesar Salad.
- Chook-N-Caesar Salad.
- All salad dressings are GF, including the Caesar.
- Drover's Platter.
- Ribs on the Barbie.
- Botany Bay Fish O'the Day.
- Chicken on the Barbie.
- House or Caesar Salad.
- Steak & Veggie Griller.
- Chicken & Veggie Griller.
- Alice Springs Chicken.
- Jackeroo Chops.
- Rockhampton Rib-Eye.
- Victoria's Filet.
- New York Strip.
- Prime Minister's Prime Rib.
- Outback Special.
- The Melbourne.
- Outback Rack.
- Add on Mates.
- Jacket Idaho Potato.
- Barbecue sauce.

Note:

- ☐ Aussie Chips are **not GF;** instead choose jacket potato or sweet potato.

- ☐ Substitute steamed vegetables (which are not GF because of seasoned mix) with steamed vegetables without seasonings, baked potato, or sweet potato.

- ☐ Be sure to request **no** croutons on salads.

- ☐ Avoid the pasta.

- ☐ Avoid the seasoned rice; it is not GF.

- ☐ Avoid Cinnamon Apples.

- ☐ Avoid the sautéed 'Shrooms.

Outback's burgers are made from 100-percent beef and the bacon, mayonnaise, mustard, ketchup, cheeses, barbecue sauce, and honey mustard sauce are all gluten-free. The grilled chicken is also gluten-free. Avoid the bread! Some restaurants will allow you to bring in your own bread. Do not send it to the kitchen though; simply order your sandwich without the bread and build it at the table. If you are unsure, call the restaurant ahead of time to ask about their policy.

Junior Menu:

- Junior ribs.
- Boomerang Cheese Burger.
- Spotted Dog Sundae.
- Sydney's Sinful Sundae.
- You can also order ice cream with chocolate sauce or homemade caramel sauce.

Again, **Aussie Chips are not GF**, so substitute vegetables without seasoning, potato, or sweet potato and avoid the bread.

To contact Outback Steakhouse go to *www.outback.com.*

Chipotle Mexican Restaurant

Everything is gluten-free except the tortillas for burritos, the soft flour tacos, and the Hot Red Tomatillo Salsa. To contact Chipotle go to *www.chipotle.com*.

This is not an all-inclusive list of restaurants that provide gluten-free foods and/or meals. This is just a sample to prove that that you can enjoy dining out even on a gluten-free diet. If you are interested in visiting a particular restaurant, do your research and investigate what it has to offer. As always, not every restaurant, even chains, will follow the same procedures. Always ask the servers and/or cooks specific questions to make sure you are ordering gluten-free foods. The information provided in this chapter can be updated at any time, so check with the companies frequently to make sure menu changes have not been made.

Websites and companies that are great resources for travel and restaurant information include:

- ☐ Good Health Publishing, LLC
  www.goodhealthpublishing.com/index.html

- ☐ What? No Wheat? Enterprises
  www.whatnowheat.com, (602) 485–8751

- ☐ CeliacTravel.com
  www.celiactravel.com/index.html

Check with your local celiac organization. Many of them have comprised lists of restaurants in *your* area that serve gluten-free meals.

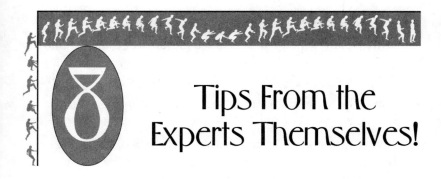

Tips From the Experts Themselves!

Helpful Hints for Living Every Day With a Gluten-free Diet

The following are tips from people who have celiac disease and live with a gluten-free diet every day. These people are experts in their own right!!

Regina Celano from Ronkonkoma, NY

- It's a good idea to find out which medications you may need, that are gluten-free, in advance. For instance, I am prone to sinus infections. Before I went to the doctor, I found out that the antibiotic Levaquin was gluten-free. If you go to the doctor unprepared, you may find yourself diagnosed and then having to do your research. It's another day or two until you get your Rx. Are you prone to ear infections, anxiety attacks, or insomnia? Make a list of gluten-free prescription medications to give to your doctor to keep in your chart and keep a copy at home, too.

- Invest in a soft-sided thermal bag with a shoulder strap and a few of the ice bags you freeze (instead of blocks, which *add* weight).

- Run, don't walk, to your local support group.

- Always, and I mean *always*, have gluten-free snacks handy in the cabinets and fridge. Carrot and celery sticks in ziplocs. String cheese and rice crackers. Bags of peanuts. Etc.

- Never be without some homemade gluten-free muffins, brownies, or other quick desserts.

- Invest in a good GF cookbook, such as Roben Ryberg's *Gluten-Free Kitchen* (Prima, 2002) and Jax Peters Lowell's *Against The Grain* (Henry Holt, 1996).

- The most important staples for the kitchen are Kinnik-Kwik Bread Mix from *www.Kinnikinnick.com*, Chebe Bread Mix from *www.Chebe.com*, and Gluten-Free Pantry Mixes for sandwich bread, muffins, and brownies from Gluten-Free Pantry (*www.gluten-free.com*); many health-food and grocery stores carry them now. All of these staples have various uses and you can never have enough on hand so stock up.

- Don't worry. There are people to help and it will get easier!

Kit Kellison from Chesapeake, VA

- Take your cell phone to the grocery store to call manufacturers about the contents of their foods. You will likely be annoyed enough while trying to find safe food and will find the will to do so. State that you have celiac disease and that you get severe damage from eating food with gluten in it, and ask if *any* gluten is added to their product. Asking whether something is "gluten-free" is not enough; something may have a small amount of gluten and still be considered "gluten-free." Remember: Every time you call a manufacturer, it takes up someone's time and costs someone money. This is important because, if enough time is wasted fielding consumer's phone calls about the allergens in products, the more likely a company will be to address this issue on labels! However, be polite and concise during your inquiries. Send e-mails or snail mail if they don't print their phone numbers on their labels.

- Join the DelphiForum Online Support Group (*forums. delphiforums.com/celiac/*). It has the most up-to-date list of member-verified safe foods, a wonderful gourmet cook who contributes daily, and members who are doctors who have the disease or have children who have the disease. It offers the ability to communicate to hundreds of other people with celiac disease about a range of topics and has been found indispensable by many grateful people who have celiac disease.

- Download medical studies to give to all healthcare providers with whom you may come in contact. Everyone from dentists who spot dental enamel defects to doctors of other specialties can be instrumental in getting someone diagnosed. Two weeks after I brought information to my endocrinologist, she told me about positive sera results for celiac disease on two of her patients. Boy, were their GIs embarrassed!

- Get a good set of knives, and learn how to use them. I often cook from scratch three times a day, so I have gotten nearly as fast as a sous chef when prepping for meals. A good, sharp, heavy, chef knife is easier to control than a little paring knife when cutting the many veggies and fruits prepared in a celiac kitchen. It is much easier to clean one knife than it is to clean all the parts of your food processor.

- Place a standing order at Kinnikinnick (*www.kinnikinnick.ca*), which automatically ships my breads, cookies, donuts, and muffins every two weeks so my kids don't have to go without. This also helps my children learn self-discipline; if they aren't careful to eat reasonable portions of goodies, they pay the consequences by having to wait for the next shipment.

- Get rid of, or segregate, all pre-GF Teflon, dishcloths, wooden spoons, wooden cutting boards, toasters, and iron skillets. All of these things are absorbent and can contaminate the things a person with celiac disease eats or eats with. Use paper towels to clean up in the kitchen so gluten isn't spread to other dishes. Better yet, keep a GF kitchen. Everyone will eat more healthy, and the non-celiacs can enjoy their pizzas and hamburgers while out of the house. I had to resort to this when I realized my teenagers were spreading crumbs throughout the house whenever I was not there to monitor their activities. Not surprisingly, I no longer have unexplained bouts of nausea and diarrhea!

- Always keep corn flour, potato flour, or potato starch on hand. I use corn flour for breading because, unlike other GF flours, it will allow the meat to become cooked before the coating burns to a hard black shell. Potato flour or starch is the best thickener for soups, sauces, and gravies. A supply of crushed GF cornflakes and GF breadcrumbs in the freezer will make life much easier should you need them.

Jessica Duvall from Williamsburg, KS

- Be a self-advocate. Don't sit by and rely on others to provide you with the information you need. Seek it and you will be empowered.

- When you cook a meal, cook an extra portion to freeze for those times when you need a "quick" dinner. (This works well for me because I am a college student).

- Build a network of support (family, friends, other people with celiac disease, Internet, books, etc.).

- Stay strong; you will have good days and bad days. Just remember that God only gives us what we can handle.

Marcy Thorner from New Market, MD

- Keep a notebook or computer file of manufacturer contacts. Include their phone numbers and dates of contact for each product. It's a good idea to schedule rechecks periodically on products that you use frequently.

- Check with the host of a children's birthday party to find out what he or she is planning to serve. Send a similar GF item for your child. If you can't stay to help serve and supervise, make special arrangements ahead of time with the host or plan to show up at serving time. Volunteer to provide the ice cream and make it a GF brand. Ask that the host set aside a serving in a separate container so as to eliminate the risk of contamination from serving spoons/scoops contacting cake.

- Always send a snack bag with a GF child for a play date, and include items that can be shared, such as microwave popping corn, fresh fruit/raisins, and cheese sticks. A child with celiac disease will feel less isolated if his or her snacks are acceptable to non-GF playmates.

- Help teach young children with celiac disease to make good food choices very early by labeling pantry and refrigerator items that are GF with a fun sticker. Tell the child, *"You can help yourself to the things with the Spiderman sticker, but the others will make you sick."*

- Come up with a catchy way to refer to your child's GF foods. If the child's first name is Allison, for example, call it "Special Allison Food" and use the acronym "SAF."

- Enlist the aid of older children (playmates, cousins, and so forth) to help supervise at family gatherings or parties. Don't convey a ton of responsibility, but suggest that they come and get you right away if they see your child reaching for the cookies, cake, and so on.

- Keep a GF grill and a separate toaster for GF bread.

- Don't use wooden spoons or cutting boards.

- Enlist the aid of GF children in determining whether certain foods are acceptable. Start them reading labels very young, and be patient when they struggle with difficult words. Engage children in being proactive, in making good decisions, and in acquiring knowledge about what is healthy for them. Start early to make it a lifelong habit.

- Keep it simple when ordering at restaurants. Mention "celiac disease" by name, just in case the server might be knowledgeable, but don't count on that to communicate your needs. *"My daughter* (or I), *have celiac disease, which is like a food allergy...."* Most people understand that food allergies can have dire consequences, and that should be adequate to engage them in helping to safeguard your child's health or your health. If not, don't hesitate to ask for the manager or chef.

- If at all possible, call ahead when you are planning to dine out. Let a manager or chef know that you will be needing some special assistance. Tell him or her when you are coming and discuss menu items that may be suitable.

- I like Bette Hagman's flour mix. I often add a few tablespoons of bean flour and/or cornstarch to the mix (replacing an equal amount). My impression is that the more flours used in a blend, and the less plain rice flour used, the better.

- Look for recipes that use very little flour. I would always select a torte recipe (many use no flour or only a few tablespoons) over a regular cake recipe (that calls for a couple of cups).

Miki Ruffino from Destrehan, LA

- I like to keep lots of fresh fruit on hand, washed and ready to eat in sealable bags. Orville Redenbacher Natural Popcorn for the microwave is another handy snack.

- When I first found out I had celiac disease it was absolutely all I could think about. But time heals that initial shock and then we settle into the everyday routine. It is like any other major change I made. After 21 days it becomes a habit.

Lila Brendel from Bismarck, ND

- I put a red sticker on my gluten-free items after I purchase them so my family knows they are gluten-free (for example, the butter, jelly, peanut butter). Also, after I read labels of common foods and find them gluten-free, I put a sticker on them so I don't have to reread the ingredients. I also do this if I make a gluten-free casserole with pasta and freeze it.

- I order pasta, snacks, and flour in large quantities (to save on shipping) and freeze them.

- I always have a container of GF powder cream soup mix and GF Bisquick mix on hand in the freezer.

- I use tomato juice in place of tomato soup in casseroles and thicken with minute tapioca or Knox gelatin.

- Keep baking potatoes on hand to either warm and add favorite toppings or slice and dry.

Pat Bridges from Welland, ON Canada

- If you aren't 100-percent sure, don't eat it.

- I never go anywhere without packing either my small or large cooler (depending on the length of the trip) with non-perishable foods and drinks, including cutlery, serviettes, and cups.

- Don't let other people's negative attitudes get to you. You know what's best. If they can't deal with it, so be it.

Anonymous Contributer

- Read labels, reread labels, and then read labels again. Many companies change ingredients frequently. Know what to look for on your label. Know the key words.

- Always ask questions in restaurants and everyone's home— even your own parents' home, after 50 years.

- Always be polite, grateful, and gracious.

- Think of what you *can* eat, not what you *cannot* eat.

Connie Rieper from Fayetteville, AR

- Don't be afraid to experiment.

- Rice cooks at low temperatures. Rice flour does cook best at lower oven temps (250–300 degrees). If the outside of your food cooks (or burns) and the inside is wet, then the cooking temperature is too high!

Jason Estes from Fayetteville, AR

- Just because it's meat doesn't mean it is gluten-free (referring to additives, preservatives, and flavorings).

Wendy Percival from Kansas City, MO

- At children's schools, I have kept frozen GF cupcakes in the nurse's freezer, kept a box of GF candy choices in the classroom, or even sent something special when I knew there would be a treat in the classroom.

- At birthday parties I usually ask if I can send along a plate of GF brownies or something so that my kids can share with the other guests as well. If there will be pizza, sometimes we bring our own along or eat before we go. Often, if I explain our circumstances, the hosts are happy to provide a snack my kids can eat.

Kristine Green from Woodlawn, TN

- I keep my most-used recipes and ingredient lists for mixes on my refrigerator for quick reference.

- I store all flours and starches in the refrigerator or freezer to help them last longer and to save cabinet space.

- I convert really short simple recipes to gluten-free and always look for already gluten-free recipes in my other cookbooks.

- For college students, instead of purchasing a food token, book, or card to eat at the cafeteria, take that money and put it into an account at a bank nearby. Use that account to order gluten-free foods throughout the year. Set it up so that only certain amounts of money can come out as orders and as cash per day. The cash can be used for drinks, fruits, or snacks on campus. This way the money is only used for food, and no worries of cross contamination. If orders are made every so many days, instead of all at once, then storage won't be an issue. There are post offices on most campuses for the students, so delivery isn't an issue either. Some areas have local support groups where you might find people nearby who could allow you to come by and heat up something or store gluten free foods for you. It never hurts to ask. You can offer to clean, do chores, or do computer work for a group for payment. Just be creative to save time, money, and mainly pain.

Rolf Meyersohn from New York City, NY

- Don't feel sorry for yourself! Remember: You can eat everything except foods that contain gluten.

- We are finally leaving the Dark Ages of prescribed foods. We can drink Scotch, we can eat pickles, and we don't have to fear blue cheese or gorgonzola. Best of all, we can begin to rely on real scientists and real research, instead of counter phobic threats and dire warnings. I suggest reading Dr. Kasarda's contributions on *www.celiac.com*; and you should certainly subscribe to *Gluten Free Living* (PO Box 105, Hastings, NY 10706.)

- For most dishes you really don't need a special GF cookbook and can rely on the great basic cookbooks (including Christopher Kimball's *The Cook's Bible*.) But of course, for baked goods, you do need special recipes. I bake bread based on recipes from Bette Hagman's *The Gluten-Free Gourmet Bakes Bread* as well as the more recent collection by Karen Robertson, *Cooking Gluten-Free*.

- When you are in a restaurant, it is probably easier to tell the waiter and chef that you have an *allergy*, rather trying to explain the problems of celiac disease. The concept of allergy and the dire consequences of trespassing its restrictions are widely understood. Besides, at some level, it's true.

- Use the Internet. The listserv *maelstrom.stjohns.edu/archives/celiac.html* might have more stuff than you need, but it deals with necessities—as well as luxuries. Recently, for example, I learned about the greatest place in the world for macaroons: *www.stjulienmacaroons.com*.

- When you leave the house in the morning, take crackers. The ones I have settled on are called *Fette Tostate*, made in Italy by Bi-Aglut. They cost $3.95 a box and can be ordered from various Websites, including *www.glutensolutions.com*. I prefer WASA Gluten-free crackers, but they are very hard to find.

Barbara Westmoreland from Hampstead, NH

- Find a doctor and nutritionist who specialize in celiac disease.

- Get on the Internet. Start with *www.celiac.com* and read about the illness. Go to the support group section and get the number of the group nearest you. Call ASAP and get yourself a local mentor.

- Find treats to have when others are indulging in glutinous foods. I have shrimp cocktail and nuts as favorites. Chips are good munchies. Find allowable candies. My spirits soared when I found Russell Stover's chocolates on a GF list. Also when I found that all Just Born candies are GF. Find and purchase treats just for you.

- When starting out, revise the home kitchen. Go through and mark everything as good, bad, or unknown. I used green, red, and yellow stickers from Staples. Separate the red from the green. If possible, go strictly gluten-free. It's so much easier knowing that if it's there, it's edible for all. Give forbidden foods to celiac-free friends. Stock up on gluten-free products, especially things you always have in the kitchen, such as ketchup and mayonnaise, using the lists as guides. Call companies and ask about the gluten status of the unknown products. Fill the flour canister with an all-purpose GF mix.

- Subscribe to the *St. John's Celiac Listserv* (a bimonthly publi-cation) and read every day. I created a folder in my Yahoo mail system, and I send the messages to the appropriate folder if I want to keep it for reference.

- Attend any and all workshops and conferences on the sub-ject of celiac disease and gluten-free diets. There is so much to learn. The sooner you get the required amount of edu-cation, the sooner you'll learn to live well with celiac dis-ease and take the diet in stride.

- Subscribe to celiac newsletters.

- Order some cookbooks and start experimenting. Always plan to make two things on any given day, because when you have one for the garbage and one for you, your celebration of the successful one overrides the disappointment in the other. If you only have one, and it goes to the garbage, you're bound to end up in tears. And remember: Every success you have is one more thing that you can safely eat for the rest of your life. It's not a today treat. It's a forever food. Make sure you take good care of the recipe.

- Give back. Talk about it and say the words: celiac, gluten-free, no wheat, rye, barley, or oat products, please. Help us get this disease out of the closet and into the public eye. Celiac disease is the most underdiagnosed chronic condition in America. There are so many people out there who would become healthy again, if properly diagnosed. At the stores and restaurants, "Gluten-free? Where is it? We want it. There are many of us, and it would be worth your while to accommodate us."

- Share it. Take the next person who tearfully tells you she/he or theirs have just been diagnosed with celiac disease and give them a hug and a loaf of GF bread. Hold their hand and share your knowledge and positive attitude with them. Take them out to lunch, go shopping together. Be their lifeline until they are properly empowered. Then watch them fly and rejoice when they pass on those feelings to someone else in need. Then give yourself a big hug and wait for the next opportunity to expand your soul. It feels so good!

Teresa A. Van Nuland from Kenosha, WI
- Buy a second freezer for your garage or basement.

- Buy groceries in bulk (for example purchase 10 boxes of GF yogurt sticks at a time, freeze them).

- Bake two to three batches at a time. Bag or wrap individual serving sizes and freeze for later use.

Pingkan Lucas from Munich, Bavaria, Germany

- My saving grace was looking toward the east. Many Southeast Asian dishes (Thai, Vietnamese, Indonesian, Malaysian) are GF by nature or are easily made into GF meals. The food is delicious, easy to make, and very healthy, with a variety of vegetables, herbs and spices. This has made my life and my diet *more* than bearable.

Trisha B. Lyons, RD LD, MetroHealth Medical Center, Cleveland, OH

- The gluten status of ingredients changes. For this reason, it is important to stay current through reliable literature and organizations or by periodically visiting an experienced registered dietitian. I have counseled numerous patients who have unnecessarily eliminated certain ingredients for many years, thereby making their diet even more restrictive than is necessary.

- Before you schedule an appointment with a registered dietitian, please be certain he or she is specialized in glutn intolerance and gluten-free diets.

Christine A. Krahling from Easton, PA

- Upon diagnosis, it is essential to work with an adult or pediatric gastroenterologist and dietitian familiar with the basics of the GF diet and up-to-date on the latest developments concerning celiac disease. Don't hesitate to keep searching until you find the professional that best meets your post-diagnosis needs.

- Try to select professionals who can provide you with basic guidelines for a GF diet and refer you to the national celiac organizations, related Websites, and a support group in your community, if there is one.

- As you learn the basics of the GF diet, keep a surplus of foods on hand for last minute travel and emergencies such as power outages. These surplus foods can include rice cakes, gluten-free crackers, gelatin desserts, cereals, and pretzels.

Bonnie J. Kruszka from Newbury, OH, author of *Eating Gluten-Free with Emily*

- Search for a celiac disease support group. You may just find lifelong friends in the process!

Barbara Emch from Hubbard, OH

- I would say the hardest thing to deal with has been going to weddings, reunions, and other special occasions. It is best to call the caterer: Many times he or she can make you a GF version of what the other guests are having. Call in the early afternoon before the chef gets busy.

- Remember that many of your favorite recipes can be made GF and they are just as good and maybe better. I have successfully done this for almost all my favorite recipes. Store-bought glazed donuts and jelly donuts are something I don't think I'll ever reproduce.

- Remember to be positive. People who feel sorry for themselves are tiresome and they are not helping themselves at all.

MaryBeth Doyle from Kirtland Hills, OH

- Never feel deprived. Eat to live, don't live to eat. It will soon become second nature to prepare meals. Always travel with some GF food, it is not as readily available as other foods. The airlines never seem to understand this diet. Have your own toaster, bread machine, and tub of margarine. Clean utensils if making gluten-free sandwiches and regular sandwiches (that is, mayo, mustard, etc.) at the same time.

Margaret Sheldon from Boston, MA

- My son has had to struggle with being gluten-free and a very serious athlete. The toughest part has probably been road trips. When the team travels, we research where they'll eat, so we know our son will be able to eat as well. We send boxes ahead to hotels, he packs a George Foreman grill, and we pay for a room with a microwave.

Kirsten Klinghammer from Rescue, CA

- I can remember coming out of surgery and later being given my first meal with not one single thing on the tray that I could eat—this was after giving them a really detailed list of what was okay and what wasn't! Now, if I need to be checked into the hospital, I just bring my own food and vitamins and have my family bring me more food as needed. I would make sure the doctor okays everything, too.

Dawn Croft, RD LD from Washington, DC

- Be cautious of the items made by different manufacturers. Each manufacturer includes its own additives. People with food allergies or sensitivities must be really cautious of this.

Helpful Tips from *Glutenfreeda.com*
(Yvonne Gifford and Jessica Hale)

- There are many wonderful recipes that are naturally gluten-free. This eliminates the need to modify recipes and spend time and money searching for hard to find GF products. Consider taking advantage of polenta, quinoa, wild rice, and many other delicious naturally GF products.

- Always keep a well-stocked pantry. Make your own chicken stock by using leftover, unused chicken parts and freeze the stock in one-cup portions for convenience. It not only is better for you, but it tastes better as well.

- To improve your GF baked goods, try adding an extra egg to your recipe and substituting vegetable or canola oil for butter. In addition, when converting your favorite baked goods recipes, choose recipes that have two cups of flour or less.

Resource Guide

The resource information listed in this chapter is believed to be reliable and correct at the time and printing of this book. The author assumes no liability for any errors or recent changes in contact information. Some companies produce both gluten-free and gluten-containing foods. Though most manufactures take extra precautions to prevent cross contamination, not all of them guarantee that their products are 100-percent gluten-free. You should question each manufacturer you purchase foods from about its individual guarantee.

The following lists are far from being all-inclusive; however, these resources will help get you started and will open the door to discovering more resources:

Valuable Websites

Celiac.com: *www.celiac.com*

Celiacs, Inc.: *www.e-celiacs.org*

Clan Thompson Celiac Page:
www.clanthompson.com/day2day/day2day.htm

FinerHealth & Nutrition: *www.finerhealth.com*

Glutenfreeda.com, Inc.: *www.glutenfreeda.com*

Gluten-free.org: Website collection (mostly gluten-free): *www.gluten-free.org*

Gluten Free Drugs: *www.glutenfreedrugs.com*

Mayo Clinic: *www.mayoclinic.com*

The North American Society for Pediatric Gastroenterology, Hepatology and Nutrition (NASPGHAN): *www.naspghan.org*

PlanetCeliac.com: *www.planetceliac.com/groceries.html*

University of Maryland Center for Celiac Research: *www.celiaccenter.org*

U.S. Department of Health and Human Services/National Institutes of Health: *www.nih.gov*

USDA Nutrient Database for Standard Reference: *www.nal.usda.gov/fnic*

Cookbooks

(by author)

Carol Fenster, Ph.D.

Savory Palate, Inc.
8174 South Holly, #404
Centennial (formerly Littleton), CO 80122–4004
(800) 741–5418   Fax: (303) 741–0339
E-mail: info@savorypalate.com.
www.savorypalate.com

Gluten-Free 101: Easy, Basic Dishes without Wheat (2003)

Gluten-Free Celebrations: Memorable Meals without Wheat (2003)

Wheat-Free Recipes & Menus: Delicious Dining without Wheat or Gluten (2002)

Special Diet Solutions: Healthy Cooking without Wheat, Gluten, Dairy, Eggs, Yeast, or Refined Sugar (2001)

Food Allergy Field Guide: A Lifestyle Manual for Families (2000), Teresa Willingham

Gluten-Free Friends: An Activity Book for Kids (2003), Nancy Patin Falini, MA, RD, LDN

Bette Hagman

Henry Holt & Company
115 West 18th St.
New York, NY 10011

The Gluten-Free Gourmet Bakes Bread

The Gluten-Free Gourmet Living Well Without Wheat, Revised Edition

More From the Gluten-Free Gourmet Delicious Dining Without Wheat

The Gluten-Free Gourmet Cooks Fast and Healthy

The Gluten-Free Gourmet Cooks Dessert

Karen Robertson

Celiac Publishing
P.O. Box 99603
Seattle, WA 98199
(206) 282–4822

Cooking Gluten Free! A Food Lovers Collection of Chef and Family Recipes Without Gluten or Wheat

Roben Ryberg

Rockling, CA: Prima Publishing, 2000

The Gluten-Free Kitchen: Over 135 Delicious Recipes for People with Gluten Intolerance or Wheat Allergy

Sheri L. Sanderson

Woodbine House Publisher, 2002

Incredible Edible Gluten-Free Food for Kids

Connie Sarros

> 3270 Camden Rue
> Cuyahoga Falls, OH 44223
> (330) 929–1651
> E-mail: gfcookbook@hotmail.com
> *Wheat Free Gluten Free Cookbook for Kids and Busy Adults*:
> *www.homestead.com/gfkids/gf.html*
> *Wheat-free Gluten-free Dessert Cookbook*:
> *www.glutenfree.homestead.com/homepage.html*
> *Wheat-free Gluten-free Reduced Calorie Cookbook*:
> *www.wfgf.homestead.com/gf.html*
> *Wheat-free Gluten-free Recipes for Special Diets*

Anne Sheasby (Editor)

> Southwater Publishing, 2002
> *Gluten-Free Cooking (Eating for Health Handbooks)*

Cooking Schools/Clubs

***Glutenfreeda* Online Cooking Magazine**

> 4809 South Kip Lane
> Spokane, WA 99224
> (509) 448–9095/ (360) 378–3675   Fax (360) 378–3673
> *www.glutenfreeda.com*

The Natural Gourmet

> 48 W. 21st St., 2nd floor
> New York, NY 10010
> (212) 645–5170   Fax: (212) 989–1493
> E-mail: info@naturalgourmetschool.com
> *www.naturalgourmetschool.com*

What? No Wheat? Enterprises

4757 E. Greenway Rd., Suite 107B # 91
Phoenix, AZ 85032–8510
(602) 485–8751   Fax: (602) 485–4411
E-mail: whatnowheat@whatnowheat.com
www.whatnowheat.com

Books

Shelley Case, B. Sc., RD

Gluten-Free Diet: A Comprehensive Resource Guide, Revised Edition. (Case Nutrition Consulting, 2002)
www.glutenfreediet.ca

Good Health Publishing, LLC

Gluten/Wheat Free guide to Eating Out
www.goodhealthpublishing.com

Danna Korn

Wheat-Free, Worry-Free (Hay House, 2002)
Kids with Celiac Disease: A Family Guide to Raising Happy, Healthy, Gluten-Free Children (Woodbine House, 2001)

Bonnie J. Kruszka

Eating Gluten-Free with Emily
A story for Children with Celiac Disease
(Xlibris Publishing, 2003)
www.xlibris.com/EatingGlutenFreewithEmily.html
(888) 795–4274

Jax Peters Lowell

Against the Grain: The Slightly Eccentric Guide to Living Well Without Gluten or Wheat (Henry Holt, 1996)

Associations/Groups

American College of Gastroenterology

4900 B South 31st St.
Arlington, VA 22206
(703) 820–7400   Fax: (703) 931–4520
www.acg.gi.org

American Dietetic Association

216 W. Jackson Blvd.
Chicago, IL 60606–6995
(312) 899–0040
(800) 877–1600
www.eatright.org

Canadian Celiac Association

5170 Dixie Road, Suite 204
Mississauga, ON L4W 1E3 CANADA
(905) 507–6208   Fax: (905) 507–4673
Toll Free: (800) 363–7296
E-mail: celiac@look.ca
www.celiac.ca/index.html

Celiac Disease Foundation (CDF)

13251 Ventura Boulevard, Suite 1
Studio City, CA 91604–1838
(818) 990–2354   Fax: (818) 990–2379
E-mail: cdf@celiac.org
www.celiac.org

Celiac Sprue Association/USA, Inc. (CSA/USA)

P.O. Box 31700
Omaha, NE 68131–0700
(402) 558–0600
E-mail: celiacs@csaceliacs.org
www.csaceliacs.org

Celiac Sprue Research Foundation
P.O. Box 61193
Palo Alto, CA 94306–1193
(650) 251–9865
E-mail: help@celiacsprue.org
www.celiacsprue.org

Gluten Intolerance Group (GIG) of North America
15110 Tenth Ave. SW, Suite A
Seattle, WA 98166–0353
(206) 246–6652   Fax: (206) 246–6531
E-mail: info@gluten.net
www.gluten.net

Dietitians Specializing in Gluten-free Diets

Jean Borgia, RD CDN
United Cerebral Palsy Center
1020 Mary Street
Utica, NY 13501
(315) 724–6907, Ext. 2285
E-mail: Info@ucp-utica.org

Shelley Case, B. Sc., RD
Case Nutrition Consulting, *www.glutenfreediet.ca*
Gluten Free Diet: A Comprehensive Resource Guide
Co-Author: *Celiac Section, Manual of Clinical Dietetics, American Dietetic Association and Dietitians of Canada*
Medical Advisory Board: Celiac Disease Foundation, Gluten Intolerance Group, Canadian Celiac Association
Dietitian Advisory Board: *Gluten-Free Living* magazine

Maggie Davis, MS, RD, LD, FADA, CDE
Leslie Cordella-Simon, MEd, RD, LD, CDE
Live Nutrition
26 Wampum Drive, P.O. Box 1709
Brewster, MA 02631
(508) 896–9080   Fax: (508) 896–3399
www.livenutrition.com

Melinda Dennis, MS RD, LDN
Beth Israel Deaconess Medical Center
Nutrition Services, Rabb B06
333 Bookline Ave.
Boston, MA 02215
(617) 667–2565
E-mail: Deletethewheat@aol.com
Founder/owner of Delete the Wheat: Nutritional Counseling for the Gluten-Free Diet& General Health, she offers one-on-one shopping tours to individuals with celiac disease, as well as store-, hospital-, and community-based lectures on celiac disease and gluten-free lifestyles.

Sandra Fishman, MS RD
625 Spring Street
Wyomissing, PA 19610
(610) 374–1944
E-mail: eatwelbwel@aol.com

Karen Francis, RD, CD-N
Registered Dietitian, Certified Dietitian-Nutritionist
Right Choices Nutrition, LLC
Monroe, CT 06468
(203) 452–7036
E-mail: kdfrancis@earthlink.net
www.rightchoices-nutrition.com
"Helping People Make The Right Choices About Food & Nutrition"

Cynthia Kupper, RD, CD

Executive Director
Gluten Intolerance Group (GIG)
(206) 246–6652   Fax: (206) 246–6531
www.gluten.net

Trisha B. Lyons, RD, LD

MetroHealth Medical Center
Cleveland, OH
(216) 778–7835 (appointments)
E-mail: Tlyons@metrohealth.org

Nancy Mazarin, MS, RD, CNS

935 Northern Boulevard
Great Neck, New York 11021
(516) 466–9087

Jennifer McCahan, RD

Harrisburg, PA 17111
(717) 903–0155
E-mail: JenMcCahan@aol.com

Carol Rees Parrish, RD, MS

Nutrition Support Specialist
Digestive Health Center of Excellence
University of Virginia Health System
Charlottesville, VA
(434) 924–8167
E-mail: crp3a@virginia.edu

Jan Patenaude, RD

Consultant Dietitian available for telephone and distance
consultations
(970) 963–3695

Jan Patenaude, RD

c/o LEAP program (Lifestyle, Eating and Performance)
Signet Diagnostic Corporation
3444 Fiscal Court, Suite #8–9
Riviera Beach, FL 33404
(888) Now–LEAP (toll free)
(888) 669–5327

Elaine Weyant, MS RD LD

Registered Dietitian
Memorial Hermann Hospital Southeast
Houston, Texas
(281) 929–6222   Fax: (281) 929–4118

Andrea Yoder, RD

Clinical Nutritionist
Digestive Health Center of Excellence
University of Virginia Health System
Charlottesville, VA
(434) 982–2565
E-mail: ajy4b@virginia.edu

American Dietetic Association

Find a Dietitian
www.eatright.org/find.html

Sub-Group of American Dietetic Association

Dietitians specializing in gastrointestinal disorders
E-mail: DIGIDRDs@aol.com

Support Groups

Raising Our Celiac Kids (R.O.C.K)

National Celiac Disease Support Group
Danna Korn
3527 Fortuna Ranch Road
Encinitas, CA 92024
(858) 395–5421
E-mail: danna@celiackids.com
www.celiackids.com

Find a support group in your area:

www.enabling.org/ia/celiac/#support

GFCF (Gluten Free Casein Free Diet) Diet Support Group

www.gfcfdiet.com

Message Boards/List Servs

Celiac.com Message Board

www.celiac.com

Delphiforums

Celiac Disease Online Support Group
forums.delphiforums.com/celiac

Maelstrom…An Internet Resource Contributed by St. John's

Celiac/Coeliac Wheat/Gluten-Free List
celiac@maelstrom.stjohns.edu
maelstrom.stjohns.edu/archives/celiac.html

Newsletters/Publications

Celiac.com's Guide to a Scott-Free Life Without Gluten (Newsletter):

E-mail: info@celiac.com
www.celiac.com

Gluten-Free Living

A quarterly magazine for people with Gluten Sensitivity.
Ann Whelan, founder and editor/publisher of Gluten-Free
Living
P.O. Box 105
Hastings-on-Hudson, NY 10706
(914) 969–2018
E-mail: gfliving@aol.com
www.glutenfreeliving.com

Glutenfreeda Online Cooking Magazine

4809 South Kip Lane
Spokane, WA 99224
(509) 448–9095/ (360) 378–3675   Fax: (360) 378–3673
www.glutenfreeda.com

Sully's Living Without, Inc.

P.O. Box 2126
Northbrook, IL 60065
(847) 480–8810
E-mail: Subscriptions@LivingWithout.com
www.livingwithout.com

Travel

Glutenfreeda OnlineCooking Magazine

4809 South Kip Lane
Spokane, WA 99224
(509) 448–9095/ (360) 378–3675   Fax: (360) 378–3673
www.glutenfreeda.com

1-888-Inn-Seek

www.1-888-inn-seek.com/GFinns.htm

Gluten-free Food Companies/Distributors

Alpineaire Foods

DG Management
P.O. Box 1799
Rocklin, CA 95677
(800) 322–6325   Fax: (916) 624–1604
E-mail: info@aa-foods.com
www.aa-foods.com

Amy's Kitchen

P.O. Box 7868
Santa Rosa, CA 95407
(707) 578–7270   Fax: (707) 570–0306
E-mail: amy@amyskitchen.net
www.amyskitchen.com

Authentic Foods

1850 W. 169th St., Suite B
Gardena, CA 90247
(310) 366–7612   Fax: (310) 366–6938
E-mail: sales@authenticfoods.com
www.authenticfoods.com

Bob's Red Mill

5209 SE International Way
Milwaukie, OR 97222
(800) 349–2173   Fax: (503) 653–1339
www.bobsredmill.com

'Cause You're Special!

Gourmet Gluten-Free Foods
P.O. Box 316
Phillips, WI 54555
(866) NO–WHEAT, (866) 669–4328 [Toll Free]
(715) 339–6959   Fax: (603) 754–0245
E-mail: Info@causeyourespecial.com
www.causeyourespecial.com

Chebe Bread

Chebe Bread Products
P.O. Box 991
Newport, VT 05855
(800) 217–9510
E-mail: info@chebe.com
www.chebe.com

Dietary Specialties

10 Leslie Court
Whippany, NJ 07981
(888) 640–2800   Fax: (973) 895–3742
E-mail: info@dietspec.com
www.dietspec.com

Eden Foods, Inc.

701 Tecumseh Road
Clinton, Michigan 49236
(888) 441–EDEN (3666)
E-mail: info@edenfoods.com
www.edenfoods.com

Ener-G Foods, Inc.

5960 First Avenue South
P.O. Box 84487
Seattle, WA 98124–5787
(206) 767–6660
(800) 331–5222   Fax: (206) 764–3398
E-mail: heidi@ener-g.com
ener-g.com

Enjoy Life Foods, LLC

Cindy R. Kaplan
1601 N. Natchez
Chicago, IL 60707
(773) 889–5070   Fax: (773) 889–5090
E-mail: ckaplan@enjoylifefoods.com
www.enjoylifefoods.com

Foods by George

3 King Street
Mahwah, NJ 07430
(201) 612–9700   Fax: (909) 279–1784

Freeda Vitamins

36 East 41st Street
New York, NY 10017
(800) 777–3737   Fax: (212) 685–7297
E-mail: FreedaVits@aol.com
www.freedavitamins.com

Gluten Evolution

(Gluten Evolution is a personal chef service completely dedicated to cooking for individuals and families who must maintain a wheat- and gluten-free diet.)

(646) 281–6247 or (319) 354–3886
Fax: (319) 358–9671
E-mail: info@glutenevolution.com
www.glutenevolution.com

The Gluten Free Cookie Jar

P.O. Box 52
Trevose, PA 19053
(888) Gluten–0   Fax: (215) 355–7991
E-mail: dsutter@glutenfreecookiejar.com
www.glutenfreecookiejar.com

Gluten-Free Delights, Inc.

P.O. Box 284
316 State St.
Cedar Falls, IA 50613
(888) 403–1806
E-mail: diana@glutenfreedelights.com
www.glutenfreedelights.com

The Gluten-Free Mall

(415) 664–4456
E-mail: info@glutenfreemall.com
www.glutenfreemall.com

The Gluten Free Market, Inc.

174 McHenry Rd
Buffalo Grove, IL 60089
(847) 419–9610   Fax: (847) 419–9615
E-mail: info@glutenfreemarket.com
www.glutenfreemarket.com

GlutenFreeMixes.Com

16004 SW Tualatin-Sherwood Road, #123
Sherwood, OR 97140
(888) 225–3432 Toll free   Fax: (503) 925–8190
E-mail: CustomerService@GlutenFreeMixes.com
www.glutenfreemixes.com

The Gluten-Free Pantry

P.O. Box 840
Glastonbury, CT 06033
Inquiries & Customer Service: (860) 633–3826
Orders Only: (800) 291–8386   Fax: (860) 633–6853
E-mail: pantry@glutenfree.com
www.glutenfree.com

Gluten-Free Trading Co., LLC

604A W. Lincoln Avenue
Milwaukee, WI 53215
(888) 993–9933   Fax: (414) 385–9915
E-mail: info@gluten-free.net
www.gluten-free.net

Gluten Solutions, Inc.

3810 Riviera Drive, Suite 1
San Diego, CA 92109
(888) 845–8836
E-mail: info@glutensolutions.com
www.glutensolutions.com

Glutino

(800) 363–DIET (3438)
E-mail: info@glutino.com
www.glutino.com

Kingsmill Foods

(416) 755–1124
E-mail: kingsmill@kingsmillfoods.com
www.kingsmillfoods.com

Kinnikinnick Foods

10940-120 Street
Edmonton, Alberta T5H 3P7 CANADA
(780) 424–2900   Fax: (780) 421–0456
Toll Free Line: (877) 503–4466
E-mail: info@kinnikinnick.com
www.kinnikinnick.ca

Miss Roben's

91 Western Maryland Parkway, Suite 7
Hagerstown, MD 21740
(800) 891–0083   Fax: (301) 665–9584
E-mail: info@missroben.com
www.missroben.com

Nutrition, Herbs & Diet

750 South 25th Street
Easton, PA 18042
(610) 252–7707
www.glutenfree4life.com

Road's End Organics, Inc.

120 Pleasant Street, E-1
Morrisville, VT 05661
Toll Free: (877) 247–3373   Fax: (802) 888–2646
E-mail: feedback@chreese.com
www.roadsendorganics.com

Twin Valley Mills, LLC

RR 1 Box 45
Ruskin, NE 68974
(402) 279–3965
E-mail: sorghumflour@hotmail.com
www.twinvalleymills.com

Don't Be Afraid to Ask!

Frequently Asked Questions and Answers

There are plenty of questions that will come up as you or a family member deals with starting a gluten-free diet. This chapter will touch on some of those questions and provide those much-needed answers.

Q. What is celiac disease?

Celiac disease is a autoimmune disorder of the small intestines that can surface at any age. People with celiac disease must avoid all foods that contain gluten, which is found in wheat, rye, barley, and its derivatives. For people with celiac disease, consuming gluten causes an autoimmune reaction that triggers the destruction of the villi within the inner lining of the small intestines. Their bodies produce antibodies that attack the small intestines, causing damage and illness.

Q. Is celiac disease genetic?

Yes, genetic factors are involved with celiac disease. It is still unclear whether a dominant or a recessive gene passes on the disease. Research shows that close relatives of a person with celiac disease have about a five- to 15-percent chance of developing the disease.

Q. Is there a cure for celiac disease?

No. There is currently no cure or drugs to treat celiac disease. However, they continue to research all possibilities. Fortunately, people with celiac disease can lead a perfectly normal and healthy life by following a strict gluten-free diet. You may require additional medical therapy for other health issues caused by celiac disease such as vitamin/mineral supplements.

Q. How common is celiac disease?

New studies indicate that celiac diseases is much more common than it was once thought to be. According to a new study by the University of Maryland Center for Celiac Research, nearly one out of every 150 Americans suffers from celiac disease. The same research also indicated that celiac disease is twice as common as Crohn's disease, ulcerative colitis, and cystic fibrosis combined.

Q. How is celiac disease treated?

Completely eliminating gluten from the diet is the only known treatment for celiac disease. A gluten-free diet is essential for life. Following a gluten-free diet means avoiding any food products that contain wheat, rye, barley, and their derivatives. Oats are questionable, so check with your doctor and dietitian.

Q. What is gluten?

Gluten is the part of flour that provides dough with its structure, provides leavening and holds products together. Gluten is a general term used for the storage proteins or *prolamins* in wheat, rye, and barley. The term *gluten-free* is used as a broad term in reference to the diet for celiac disease to describe a food or diet that is void of prolamins from wheat, rye, and barley. The part of the storage proteins that actually causes the destruction of the intestinal villi in people with celiac disease and dermatitis herpetiformis is termed "prolamins." The names of the prolamins are *gliadins* in wheat, *secalins* in rye, and *hordeins* in barley.

Q. Can I eat any amount of gluten?

No. Once on a gluten-free diet, a person with celiac disease must follow a strict gluten-free diet. Any amount of gluten in the diet can begin to cause damage to the small intestines, even if it does not present symptoms.

Q. What are the symptoms of celiac disease?

Symptoms of celiac disease vary between individuals. Common symptoms include diarrhea, abdominal pain, gas, bloating, weight loss, chronic fatigue, weakness, malnutrition, and other gastrointestinal ailments. Children may also experience failure to thrive or grow, irritability, lack of concentration, diarrhea, and bloating. People with celiac disease may also be affected by other health problems as a result of the body's inability to absorb nutrients such as osteoporosis, anemia, muscle cramping, and fatigue. They may also experience arthritis, joint pain, reproductive difficulties, depression, and behavioral changes.

Q. Do all people with celiac disease experience symptoms?

No. Some people with celiac disease may not show symptoms. They may have an undamaged part of their small intestines that is able to absorb enough nutrients to prevent experiencing some of these symptoms. However, even though they may not experience symptoms they are still at risk for the complications of celiac disease.

Q. How is celiac disease diagnosed?

A blood test is used to screen people for the presence of specific antibodies. An intestinal biopsy of the small intestines (before beginning a gluten-free diet) is performed to make the final diagnosis.

Q. What are the complications associated with celiac disease?

If left untreated, celiac disease can be life-threatening. People with celiac disease are more likely to be afflicted with health problems that are related to malabsorption (the inability to absorb nutrients into the body) including osteoporosis, osteopenia, tooth enamel defects, pancreatic disease, central and peripheral nervous system disease, internal hemorrhaging, organ disorders (gallbladder, liver, or spleen), and gynecological disorders. People who do not adhere strictly to a gluten-free diet stand a greater risk of developing certain types of cancer (lymphoma and adencarcinoma) in the intestines.

Q. Is celiac disease ever misdiagnosed as another illness or disease?

Celiac disease can be *very* difficult to diagnose because its symptoms mirror those of other gastrointestinal disorders, such as irritable bowel syndrome (IBS), Crohn's disease, ulcerative colitis, diverticulosis, intestinal infections, chronic fatigue syndrome, and depression. The average length of time from the start of symptoms and a confirmed diagnosis in the United States is 11 years. If your physician suspects celiac disease you should be referred to a gastroenterologist (a specialist in the areas of the stomach and intestines) who has experience with celiac disease.

Q. Are there other diseases related to celiac disease?

There appears to be a higher incidence of certain disorders that are related to the immune system among people who have celiac disease. Some of these include Type 1 diabetes (insulin-dependent diabetes mellitus), Graves' disease, Addison's disease, scleroderma, chronic active hepatitis, systemic lupus erythematosus, Sjogren's syndrome, Down syndrome, dermatitis herpetiformis, liver disease, kidney disease, and rheumatoid arthritis.

Q. What is dermatitis herpetiformis, and what does it have to do with gluten?

Dermatitis herpetiformis (DH) is a chronic and severe disease of the skin that presents itself with itchy skin blisters on the elbows, knees, buttocks, scalp, and back. DH is also a genetic autoimmune disease and is linked to celiac disease, though both are separate diseases. In fact, about five percent of people with celiac disease will develop DH, either before being diagnosed or within the first year on the diet. DH is also *treated* with a gluten-free diet as well as medications to control the skin rash. Most people with DH do not have obvious gastrointestinal symptoms, but almost all have some type of damage to the small intestines. Therefore they also have the potential for all of the nutritional problems of a person with celiac disease. Both celiac disease and DH are permanent and symptoms and damage will occur if gluten is consumed.

Q. What is lactose intolerance, and how is it related to celiac disease?

Lactose is a natural sugar found in milk and milk products. Lactose intolerance is a condition that stems from a lack of the enzyme (lactase) that is needed to break down the milk sugar lactose. Symptoms of lactose intolerance may include some or all of the following: bloating, gas, abdominal cramping, diarrhea, nausea, and headache. For people with celiac disease, lactose intolerance is more prevalent because the damage to the gastrointestinal tract can reduce the level of lactase in the body. Lactose intolerance is usually only temporary until the condition is under control and the small intestines heals.

Q. Is there a connection between celiac disease and diabetes?

Yes. There is a strong correlation between celiac disease and Type 1 diabetes. The prevalence of Type 1 diabetes in the general population is about 0.5 percent where in people with celiac disease it is approximately five to 10 percent. There has been no connection found between celiac disease and the more common form of Type 2 diabetes.

Q. What is a gastroenterologist?

A gastroenterologist is a physician who specializes the diagnosis and treatment of diseases and conditions of the digestive and intestinal system such as stomach pain, liver disease, diarrhea, IBS, ulcerative colitis, Crohn's disease, celiac disease, colon polyps, and cancer. They may further specialize in treating people in certain age groups such as pediatrics. Gastroenterologists can be certified by the Board of Internal Medicine, which is recognized by the American Board of Medical Specialties.

Q. This diet sounds complicated. What is the easiest way to get started?

Learning everything about a gluten-free diet can be overwhelming. There is so much to learn, remember, and look out for. But with practice it gets easier and easier until it becomes almost automatic. It basically becomes a way of life. But keep in mind to never let yourself become too complacent. Even though it may become easier, when you start to take things for granted, accidents and mistakes happen. The best way to get started is with a diet where the foods have no ingredients and are naturally gluten-free such as fresh meats, fruits, vegetables, potatoes, rice, eggs, most dairy products, and legumes. Cook your own foods and drink water and 100-percent juice. This allows you to make sure that everything you are eating is gluten-free while you are learning everything you need to learn. Also check on medications. As you begin to feel better and as you become more confident in your level of understanding of gluten-free foods and ingredients, start adding your favorite prepared foods and buying substitutes for foods that contain gluten. Take small steps so you won't feel overwhelmed and pay special attention to each item you add to your "safe list." Always enlist the help of a dietitian that specializes in celiac disease to help get you started.

Q. What resources are available to help me cope with this disease?

There are countless resources available for the newly diagnosed person with celiac disease. These include books, cookbooks, support groups (both local and national), dietitians,

Websites, GF food companies, message boards, camps, cooking classes and chat rooms. (See Chapter 9 for a listing of some of these resources.)

Q. I have been on a gluten-free diet and have not yet improved/I was feeling well but now my symptoms are back. Am I doing something wrong?

The gluten-free diet is not an easy one. It is up to the person with celiac disease to research absolutely everything he or she eats. It is important not to become complacent or laid-back about the diet. You must always be on your toes and be current with information on the foods you are eating. Food manufacturers often change their ingredients without announcing it, which means a product you may have always used and trusted can suddenly contain gluten. Watch for cross contamination in your home or anywhere that you may eat. Be extra careful in restaurants for situations such as a plain chicken breast being floured before being grilled or a burger being grilled on the same surface as the buns are warmed. Double-check your cosmetics such as lipstick and chapstick. Also check on stamps and/or envelopes that you may be licking. Be aware of both prescription and over-the-counter medication that you are taking. If you feel you are still eating a 100-percent gluten-free diet and are still having symptoms, check with your specialist. The antibody blood tests can be used to check for reactions to gluten ingested. You should also consider the possibility of other food intolerances.

Q. I am feeling better (or I never experienced obvious symptoms). How do I know if I am actually gluten-free?

Antibody blood tests can be used in following up on people with celiac disease to confirm that the diet is, indeed, free of gluten. The IgA antibodies tend to decrease quickly when a gluten-free diet is maintained. Therefore this test can be used to look for reactions to gluten. This reinforces the need to visit your specialist on a regular basis for follow-ups.

Q. I have always suffered with diarrhea; now I am constipated. Why?

Constipation can be due to a lack of fiber in the diet. Cook with whole grains whenever possible, use brown rice versus white rice, and use brown rice flour in baked goods when possible. Eat plenty of fresh fruits and vegetables as well as legumes. Drink plenty of water and exercise on a regular basis. If you are still having problems with constipation, speak with your specialist.

Q. Can I drink alcoholic beverages?

Some are safe and some are not. Beer, ale, and lager most definitely should be avoided because they contain malt (usually from barely) as an ingredient. Wine, sparkling wine, champagne, cognac, grappa, sherry, sake, and distilled liquors such as gin, light rum (check spiced and dark rums), tequila, vodka, scotch whiskey, and vermouth are usually safe. Some to question include wine coolers and alcoholic cider products. Most people with celiac disease will not have problems with certain distilled alcohols or vinegars, regardless of their source, because the distillation process removes gluten. If you are unsure about any alcoholic product check the ingredient list. Always drink alcoholic beverages responsibly.

Q. Is wheat-free the same thing as gluten-free?

No. Wheat-free is *not* the same thing as gluten-free. Wheat-free products may have no wheat, but they could still contain rye or barley, which are both gluten-containing ingredients.

Q. Are there tax deductions for the purchases of special gluten-free foods?

Tax deductions for gluten-free foods can be used as medical expenses on your taxes. You can deduct the difference between the cost of the gluten-containing food and the extra cost, if any, of the gluten-free food. The full cost of any special items needed for a gluten-free diet can be deducted, such as guar or xanthan gum. You can deduct the cost of the trips you make to gluten-free specialty stores. You can also deduct the full cost of postage or other delivery expenses on gluten-free purchases that you make. Make sure you have a letter from your doctor indicating that you have celiac disease and must strictly follow a gluten-free diet for life in case you are ever audited. You will also need to save all proof of purchases such as receipts, registered receipts, or canceled checks for any purchases you are deducting. The total amount of your deductions for gluten-free foods and materials should be added to your other medical expenses. Do not send your doctor's letter or proof of purchases with your tax forms. You should save those documents, which would only have to be submitted in the event the IRS audits you. If you have any questions regarding medical tax deductions, speak to a certified public accountant.

Q. Is buckwheat gluten-free?

Pure buckwheat *is* gluten-free. Buckwheat (or kasha) is not wheat even though it has the word *wheat* in its name. It is classified as a fruit, not a cereal grain, and comes from a plant that is closely related to rhubarb. It is important to purchase pure buckwheat because some buckwheat mixes, flours, and pastas are made up of a mixture of buckwheat and wheat flour. Buckwheat is high in fiber and a good source of protein as well as B-vitamins, potassium, phosphorus and iron. It can be purchased in most health food stores. You can buy buckwheat raw (light), roasted (dark), or boxed and ground as a cereal. You can also buy it as noodles (soba), but check that it does not contain any wheat.

Q. Can I eat oats?

Recently research has found that some people with celiac disease can safely eat moderate amounts of uncontaminated oats without it doing any harm. However, some experts still have doubts about the safety of oats. Their concern is that even if the oat prolamin, *avenin*, is not harmful, oats can still become contaminated with wheat before reaching the consumer because the same equipment may be used for both wheat and oats. For now, the extent of the contamination of commercial oat products is not known. It is up to you, your dietitian, and your physician whether to include oats in your diet. If you do consume oats, consume only uncontaminated oat products and limit your consumption to 1/2 cup of dry, whole-grain, rolled oats (or the equivalent) per day.

Q. How important is it for a confirmed celiac to have repeat biopsies or blood tests when on a gluten-free diet?

It is very important to visit your physician on a regular basis and have blood tests. These types of tests can provide a strong indicator of whether you are strictly following a gluten-free diet and whether the gluten-free diet being followed is effective. Sometimes a person with the best intentions of following the diet can be taking a medication or some other intake that is contaminated with gluten and not realize it. This can continue the disease process. Medical professionals agree that once there is a positive diagnosis of celiac disease, the person on a gluten-free diet should have repeat blood tests after three to six months. A repeat biopsy is not necessary at this time.

Q. Can products, which contain gluten but only touch the skin, affect people with celiac disease?

Very few people with celiac disease are likely to have any type of reaction to a topical contact with a gluten-containing product. In order for a gastrointestinal reaction to occur, direct contact with gluten is required. In rare cases, topical gluten breathed into the upper airways can cause allergic rhetinitis type symptoms.

Q. How much gluten is in the normal person's diet, and how much does it take to cause damage to a celiac?

The average person's diet contains about 10 to 40 grams of gluten per day. As a point of reference, the average slice of whole-wheat bread contains about 4.8 grams of gluten, and the amount in a serving of pasta is about 6.4 grams. Basically *any* amount of gluten can cause damage in a person with celiac disease.

Q. How much wheat can be in a communion wafer?

Most communion wafers are made from wheat. Alternatives can be used in protestant churches, such as rice-based wafers, but the Catholic Church is more strict. According to the Catholic Church, the bread used in the Eucharist must be made exclusively from wheat. However, Catholics can be given permission to use a low-gluten host made from Codex wheat starch, which contain approximately 0.0374 milligrams of gluten. These are the only products currently produced that meet all of the Catholic Church's requirements. The problem is that these hosts are not 100-percent gluten-free. The Catholic Church in general recommends that worshippers with celiac disease in the United States only receive communion in the form of consecrated wine. Whether you will be allowed to use a rice-based or low-gluten product will depend on your local church. Talk to officials at your church to learn your options.

Q. Do I really need to get another toaster?

That depends on how careful you and other members of your family are. You can designate a slot for just your bread and ask everyone to thoroughly clean the toaster after using it, but if you can't rely on this to happen every time then you are safer spending the money to get yourself a small toaster.

Q. Does the gluten survive in fryer oil? If so, does it penetrate into food that would otherwise be gluten-free?

Yes. Gluten can survive in fryer oil and can contaminate gluten-free foods that are cooked in the same oil as gluten-containing foods.

Q. Does breastfeeding have any effect on the onset of celiac disease in infants?

According to a study reported in the *American Journal of Clinical Nutrition*, continuing to breastfeed infants while beginning to introduce them to certain foods may reduce their risk of developing celiac disease. The study found a much lower risk of celiac diseases in infants who were still being breastfed than in infants who were no longer breastfeeding at the time when gluten-containing foods were introduced into their diet. According to the report on this study, the risk of celiac disease was reduced by almost 40 percent in children age 2 or younger if they were still being breastfed when gluten was introduced into the diet. The chances increased even more for infants who were continued on breastfeeding after gluten was introduced. The risk for celiac disease appeared to increase when gluten-containing foods were introduced in large amounts into an infant's daily diet. More research still needs to be done.

Q. Can a woman with celiac disease who is on a gluten-free diet expect to have a normal pregnancy and delivery?

Yes. If the nutritional status of the woman is good, there are no additional health problems or risk factors, and she takes care of herself, the risk factors should be no greater than that of a woman without celiac disease.

Q. Is there any way for the average consumer to test foods for gluten besides just looking at ingredient lists?

Presently there is not, but scientists in Europe are currently developing a biosensor for the detection of gluten in food. The goal of their project is to develop a disposable system that would analyze gluten in food samples. It would allow people to conduct on-the-spot testing of fresh, cooked, or industrially processed foods. Their project is currently ongoing.

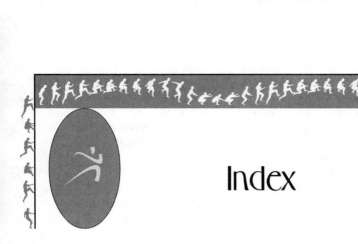

Index

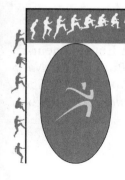

About the Author

Kimberly A. Tessmer, RD, LD
Consulting Dietitian

Kimberly has been a registered dietitian since 1992 and is also an Ohio-licensed dietitian. Her educational achievements include a Bachelor of Science in Technology (Dietetics) from Bowling State University in Bowling Green, Ohio. Kimberly currently owns and operates a consulting business called **Nutrition Focus**, in which she specializes in weight-loss services, medical nutrition therapy, authoring, and consulting.

Kimberly's current clients and endeavors, as well as her past experience as a National Corporate Dietitian for three national weight loss companies, prove her knowledge and reliability. She is the author of *The Everything Nutrition Book*. In addition, she has written numerous articles for various health/nutrition Websites and magazines such as *Bally Total Fitness* magazine, *Well and Healthy Women* magazine, *FitnessHeaven.com,* and *Healthology, Inc*. Kimberly has acted as a foodservice director and clinical dietitian for a large nursing and rehabilitation facility, where she was challenged with the task of dealing with many types of nutritional problems. She has also acted as a foodservice manager and as a dietetic technician at numerous hospitals. She is a member of the American Dietetic Association and the ADA Practice Group, Nutrition Entrepreneurs. She was recently included in the 2003–2004 Edition of the *National Register's Who's Who in Executives & Professionals*. She can be reached through her Website, *www.Nutrifocus.net*, or her e-mail, Kim@Nutrifocus.net.